Coping with Aging Series

Series Editors
John C. Rosenbek, Ph.D.
Chief, Speech Pathology and Audiology Services
William S. Middleton Memorial Hospital
Madison, Wisconsin

Medical Editor
Molly Carnes, M.D.
Department of Medicine and Institute on Aging
University of Wisconsin
Madison, Wisconsin

Associate Director for Clinical Services
Geriatric Research, Education and Clinical Center
William S. Middleton Memorial Hospital
Madison, Wisconsin

Coping with Bowel and Bladder Problems

Barbara Doherty King, M.S., RNC, GNP

Judy Harke, M.S., RNC, GNP

SINGULAR PUBLISHING GROUP, INC
SAN DIEGO, CALIFORNIA

Published by Singular Publishing Group, Inc.
4284 41st Street
San Diego, California 92105-1197

©1994 by Singular Publishing Group, Inc.

Illustrations by Loralee A. McAuliffe

Typeset in 11/14 Times by So Cal Graphics
Printed in the United States of America by McNaughton & Gunn

Library of Congress Cataloging-in-Publication Data

King, Barbara Doherty.
    Coping with bowel and bladder problems/Barbara King,
Judy Harke.
        p. cm.—(Coping with aging series)
    Includes bibliographical references and index.
    ISBN 1-56593-068-1
    1. Fecal incontinence in old age. 2. Urinary incontinence in old
    age. I. Harke, Judy. II. Title. III. Series.
RC866.D43K54   1994
618.97'6342—dc20   94-17284
                                                                   CIP

❖ Table of Contents

❖ Foreword

The books in the *Coping with Aging Series* are written for men and women coping with the challenges of aging, and for their families and other caregivers. The authors are all experienced practitioners; doctors, nurses, social workers, psychologists, pharmacists, nutritionists, audiologists, physical and occupational therapists, and speech-language pathologists.

The topics of individual volumes are as varied as are the challenges that aging may bring. These include: hearing loss, low vision, depression, sexual dysfunction, immobility, intellectual impairment, language impairment, speech impairment, swallowing impairment, death and dying, bowel and bladder incontinence, stress of caregiving, giving up independence, medications, and stroke. The volumes themselves, however, share common features. Foremost, they are practical, jargon-free, and responsible. Each contains professionally valid information translated into language people who are not health care providers can understand. Each contains useful advice and sections to help readers decide how they are doing and whether they need to do more, do less, or do something different. Each includes lists of services, suppliers, and additional readings. Each provides evidence that no single person need cope alone.

None of the volumes can substitute for appropriate professional health care. However, when combined with the care, instruction, and counseling that health care providers supply, they make coping with aging easier. America is greying at the same time its treasury is inadequate to meet its population's needs. Thus the *Coping with Aging Series* offers help for people who need and want to help themselves.

This volume, *Coping with Bowel and Bladder Problems*, is written by two geriatric nurse practitioners, both with a particular interest in problems with bowel and bladder function. Barbara King has had over 10 years experience working with older adults and their families and providing consultation and training to both professionals and nonprofessionals involved in geriatrics. She is currently at the University of Wisconsin where she is a nurse practitioner in the Geriatric Clinic and a clinical instructor in the School of Nursing. Judy Harke has worked with incontinent patients and their families for over 10 years and is currently a nurse practitioner in the Geriatrics Clinic at the University of Wisconsin where she is also a clinical specialist in the School of Nursing.

If you or someone you know is having difficulty with bowel or bladder function, this book will help you learn-about your problems, tell you where you can find assistance, and what you can do to promote normal bowel and bladder function.

John C. Rosenbek, Ph.D.
Series Editor

Molly Carnes, M.D.
Medical Editor

❖ Preface

Bowel and bladder problems, such as incontinence of urine and stool, are prevalent in the elderly, but are *not* considered normal aging. Urinary incontinence affects 15–30% of community-dwelling elderly and over 50% of all Americans in nursing homes. Of individuals who have incontinence, 10% will have both urinary and stool loss.

Loss of urine and/or stool has a dramatic impact on an individual's emotional and physical well-being. However, 50–70% of people with incontinence do not seek help for this problem. The reason for this is unclear. Some explanations may be: (1) They are too embarrassed; (2) They hope the incontinence is just a temporary problem and will get better over time; (3) They feel incontinence is a normal part of aging and nothing can be done; (4) They fear they may need surgery; (5) They do not perceive the incontinence to be a significant problem; (6) They are unaware of treatment options; (7) They have a poor relationship with their health care provider; and (8) They have low expectations about treatment success. Regardless of the reason, a large number of people with incontinence do not seek treatment. This is unfortunate, for many types of incontinence are easily treated and have a high success rate of cure or improvement.

Incontinence is also a very costly problem. Costs vary significantly, depending on the degree of incontinence, the care setting (e.g., home or nursing home), and the technique used to manage the wetness or soilage. It has been estimated to cost 3.26 billion dollars yearly to care for incontinent elderly residents of nursing homes and 4.8 billion dollars yearly to care for incontinent elderly adults who live in the community (1987 estimates). When compared to the cost of AIDS (1.8 billion dollars, 1987 estimates) and dementia or senility (15.1 billion dollars, 1987 estimates), the impact of incontinence on financial resources is substantial.

Coping with Bowel and Bladder Problems is written for people with involuntary loss of urine or stool and for their families, friends, and caregivers. This book will provide a thorough explanation of what incontinence is, the types of incontinence and possible causes, suggestions for seeking help, treatment options, and potential resources. Chapters will provide a description of what to expect during an incontinence evaluation, as well as information on how to learn bladder and bowel control through exercises and/or training programs. Medications used for treating incontinence will also be discussed, along with measures to maximize one's environment to maintain mobility and function for independent toileting.

Finally, there is a resource chapter to help you understand the products available for the management of incontinence and care of the skin. This is supplemented by a list of manufacturers, illustrations of some products, and information about support groups available for people with incontinence. It is the hope of the authors that the book, *Coping with Bowel and Bladder Problems*, will make life more satisfying for people who have incontinence by providing them with information and techniques to control involuntary urine or stool loss.

❖ Acknowledgments

We wish to thank our editors, Molly Carnes and Jay Rosenbeck, for their help and encouragement in the development and completion of this book; Patty Wagner for her computer assistance with developing documentation forms; our family members, Ron, Lindsey, and Amy King, Mike, Matt, and Melissa Harke for their patience and support during the writing of this manuscript; and the many older adults who came to us for aid and stimulated us to find better ways to treat urinary and fecal incontinence.

❖ Dedication

We dedicate this book to all those people who thought
they would never have control again.

Chapter 1

What Is Urinary Incontinence?

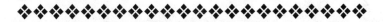

As a person ages, so does the body. Elderly people experience a decline in vision and hearing and have a higher percentage of chronic illness. Involuntary loss of urine, however, is not considered normal aging. Yet, frequently older adults and family members assume that incontinence is normal as one gets older. Additionally, family members and caregivers of the incontinent older adult may feel the individual is wetting on purpose, or for attention. Persons with incontinence may feel embarrassed about their appearance and be fearful of odor. To compensate, they may limit contacts with family and friends, avoid trips outside of their homes, and withdraw from social gatherings. Involuntary loss of urine may inhibit people from participating in enjoyable activities. Yet loss of urine is not a condition that is inevitable as people age. It is a symptom of an underlying problem and is very responsive to treatment. The first step in taking control of incontinence is to understand what it is.

What Is Urinary Incontinence?

Urinary incontinence is an involuntary loss of urine in sufficient amounts and/or sufficient frequency to be a social or health problem. For some the loss of a few drops of urine may be bothersome, whereas for others the loss is not perceived as a problem unless complete soilage of clothing occurs. Nevertheless, when the loss of bladder control becomes a problem, people will make dramatic lifestyle changes to regain control. Some examples of how people control urine loss are:

1. decrease the amount of fluids they drink;

2. seek out the location of the bathroom on a social outing, such as a shopping mall;

3. avoid travel;

4. stop attending social gatherings such as church;

5. go to the bathroom frequently; or

6. wear a pad or absorbent brief.

One woman stopped participating in her golf league because she had to toilet frequently and was afraid if she got an urge to urinate while on the golf course, she wouldn't make it to the toilet on time. Another woman avoided overnight trips and refused to travel with friends because she was afraid she would soil the bed linen.

It is unfortunate that the individuals in the examples missed out on enjoyable times with friends and family. Urinary incontinence has a high cure rate. To get a better understanding of why incontinence occurs in older adults we have to discuss the urinary system, bladder function, how aging affects the system, and other factors of aging that affect one's ability to maintain continence.

The Urinary System

The urinary system is made up of four organs: the kidneys, the ureters, the bladder, and the urethra (see the illustration on page 4). Together these structures control the function of eliminating waste from the body in the form of urine.

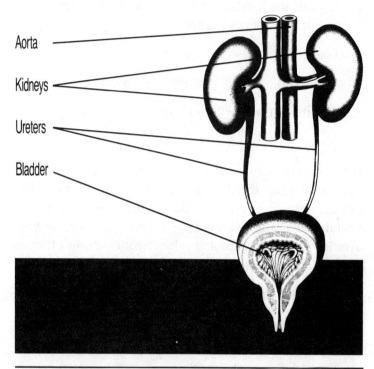

Aorta

Kidneys

Ureters

Bladder

Upper and lower urinary systems. (From *Working with the Incontinent*, a Community Education Program sponsored by DEPEND® Products. Used with permission. ®Registered Trademark of Kimberly-Clark Corp., Neenah, WI 54956. ©1986 KCC.)

The kidneys act as a colander, straining the blood and separating out what is returned to the body to use and what is eliminated as waste. The filtered waste products are combined with water to form urine. The urine flows from the kidneys to the bladder through the ureters, which are two narrow, hollow tubes.

The bladder is a muscular organ with two functions. It stores the urine produced by the kidneys and then it disposes of the urine from the body. When the bladder becomes full, it contracts and empties the urine. This process is called urinating, or voiding.

The urine leaves the bladder through the urethra. The urethra is another narrow tube that connects the bladder to the outside of the body. The opening for the urethra is at the end of the penis for men and just above the vagina for women (see the illustration on page 6).

The pelvic muscles, also called perineal muscles, are a large band of muscles that form a sling and support the pelvic organs, which consist of the bladder, urethra, and bowel, and, in women, the vagina and uterus (see the illustration on page 7) The pelvic muscles can be voluntarily contracted and relaxed to control the passage of urine from the urethra.

Bladder Function

Bladder control depends on the nervous system, which has both automatic responses for emptying the bladder, as well as a mechanism for voluntary control, allowing the individual to decide when to start or stop urination. The nerve pathways for the bladder travel through the spinal cord to the brain (see the illustration on page 8). At the base of the brain is a small area called the pons. The pons receives the signals from the spinal cord and sends it to a higher portion of the brain called the cortical control center, or micturition center. It is from the corti-

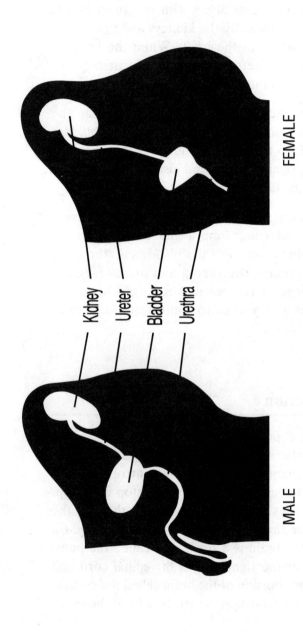

Kidney

Ureter

Bladder

Urethra

MALE

FEMALE

Lower urinary tract in men and women. (From *Working with the Incontinent*, A Community Education Program sponsored by DEPEND® Products. Used with permission. ®Registered Trademark of Kimberly-Clark Corp., Neenah, WI 54956. ©1986 KCC.)

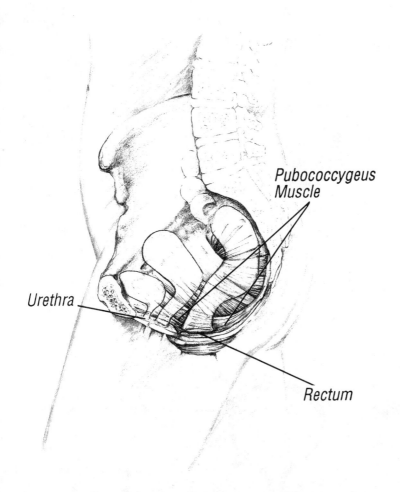

Perineal muscles.(From *Working with the Incontinent*, A
Community Education Program sponsored by DEPEND®
Products. Used with permission. ®Registered Trademark of
Kimberly-Clark Corp., Neenah, WI 54956. ©1986 KCC.)

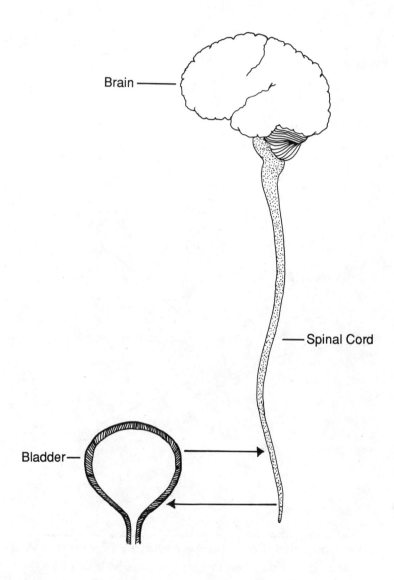

Nervous system for bladder control.

cal control center that signals are sent to the bladder to tell it to contract and empty.

As children learn to toilet train, they learn to delay the signal from the cortical control center, thereby putting off urination until they can reach a toilet. Children also learn to contract the pelvic muscles to increase the resistance in the urethra to prevent leakage of urine. Continence, therefore, is a learned process, and part of the treatment for incontinence is reestablishing control over the cortical control center.

By the time children reach adulthood, they pretty much take for granted the ability to control bladder function. Most adults empty their bladder four to eight times in a 24-hour period. Many adults do not have to void during the night. However, beyond age 65 it can be considered "normal" to get up to urinate one to two times at night. In addition, many medications, such as diuretics and blood pressure medicines, can cause night time voidings.

On the average, the adult bladder can hold 300 to 600 cubic centimeters or 10 to 20 ounces of urine. Leakage should not occur even if the need to urinate is delayed.

The Aging Bladder

Changes occur in the urinary system as people age. It is thought that these changes may make an elderly person more prone to incontinence. Some of the aging changes that occur are:

1. a decrease in the amount of urine the bladder can hold;

2. an increase in uncontrolled contractions of the bladder muscle;

3. a decrease in the ability to delay voiding; and

4. a decrease in flexibility of the bladder muscle resulting in incomplete emptying.

In women after menopause there is a decrease in estrogen. Estrogen has a direct effect on the tissue that lines the urethra and vagina. The decline of estrogen causes the tissue of the urethra and vagina to become thinner, drier, and less firm, and can make the vagina and urinary system more susceptible to infection. These changes also decrease the ability of the urethra to close tightly to prevent leakage.

As men age, the prostate gland (see the illustration on page 11) enlarges and can block or obstruct the urethra, making it more difficult to empty the bladder. The buildup of urine in the bladder eventually causes frequent dribbling of urine. This form of incontinence will be discussed in more detail in Chapter 2.

In addition to changes in the urinary system as an individual becomes older, there is also an increased likelihood of developing chronic illness. Chronic illness can have a big impact on an older adult's ability to maintain continence. People who suffer from stroke, Parkinson's disease, arthritis, or hip fracture may have a decline in their ability to walk or get out of a chair. If mobility is affected, it is more difficult to get to the toilet in a timely manner. Older adults with congestive heart failure or chronic swelling of the legs and ankles will have to urinate more frequently at night. In addition, medications may be prescribed to manage a chronic illness. Some of

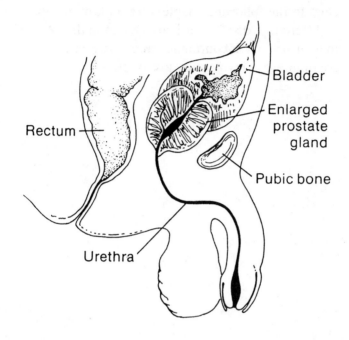

Prostate gland. (From *Nursing for Continence*, 1990, by K. Jeter, N. Fuller, and C. Norton, Philadelphia, W. B. Saunders. Reprinted with permission.)

these medications may affect the urinary tract and increase the possibility of incontinence. Specific medications that could affect bladder control will be reviewed in Chapter 2.

Summary

We have discussed how the bladder and urinary system work and changes that occur in the urinary system with aging. In the following chapters we look more closely at the different parts of the urinary system to define specific types of urinary incontinence and possible methods to cure or improve involuntary loss of urine.

Chapter 2

Narrowing Down
the Causes

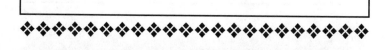

Acute Incontinence

As was noted in the previous chapter, the body changes associated with aging do not cause incontinence. Rather, they make the body less resilient and more prone to urine loss. Often the loss of control is temporary and, once the initiating factor is corrected, control is regained. The temporary loss of urine control is termed *acute incontinence*. Factors that can be associated with acute incontinence—medications, alcohol, illness, irritants, constipation, estrogen loss—are listed in the chart on page 15. It is important to consider each factor and what changes are feasible when evaluating the loss of urine control. Some factors can be adjusted independently, others need the advice of a physician or nurse.

Medications

As people age, they often need medication for chronic problems that develop. Several of these medications can decrease the ability to control urination by their effects on the bladder muscle, the bladder outlet, the nerve pathways, or on the amount of urine being produced. Medications that can interfere with bladder control include diuretics (water pills), blood pressure medications, tranquilizers, and sleeping pills. If a medication is suspected of contributing to incontinence, it should not be stopped without first consulting the person who prescribed it. When a medication is essential for health and cannot be stopped, sometimes adjustments can be made to decrease its effects on bladder control. These concerns should be discussed with a health care professional.

Factors Associated with Acute Urinary Incontinence

Medications	Diuretics
	Blood pressure medications
	Tranquilizers
	Muscle relaxants
	Sleeping pills
Alcohol	
Illness	Diabetes
	Congestive Heart Failure
	Venous Insufficiency
Irritants	Bladder infection
	Caffeine
	Nutrasweet
	Poor fluid intake
Constipation	
Estrogen loss	after menopause

Alcohol

Alcohol consumption has many effects on bladder function. It causes urgency and frequency which make it more difficult to control the bladder. It also causes sedation, which decreases one's ability to recognize bladder signals and respond in a timely manner. A 2- to 3-week trial without alcohol will help determine if this is a factor in urine loss.

Illness

A new onset of illness can affect control of urination because it adds stress to the balance of the body and upsets normal function. The additional load can decrease one's ability to think clearly, disrupting one's recognition and response to bladder signals. An individual may also have more difficulty getting to the toilet without help. New medications to treat the illness can also play a role. These combined factors increase the potential for loss of bladder control during acute episodes of illness.

There are also specific illnesses that make a person more prone to urine loss. One example is diabetes. When the blood sugar is high, the volume and frequency of urination are increased. For some people, this change is enough to initiate loss of control of urination. Whatever the underlying mechanism, often when the illness is resolved or stabilized, so is the problem with urinary incontinence.

Irritants

The bladder muscle in the older person appears to be more sensitive to irritants in the urine. The muscle becomes more hyperactive, and the individual is less able to stop it from emptying. A common irritant is urinary tract infection. Sometimes loss of urine control is the only sign a person has to indicate that a bladder infection is present. Other symptoms of a bladder infection might be: (a) voiding more frequently in small amounts, (b) having increased sense of urgency—that sudden and intense need to void, (c) having burning or pain with voiding, and (d) having blood in the urine. Once the infection is treated, these symptoms disappear, and bladder control is regained.

A low fluid intake can also contribute to incontinence because the resulting urine is very concentrated and acts as an irritant on the bladder muscle. It is recommended that you drink six to eight glasses (8 ounces) of fluid each day.

Caffeine has been shown to decrease bladder control, though it is uncertain whether it acts as an irritant to the bladder muscle or merely increases urinary frequency. Coffee, tea, soda pop, and chocolate are major sources of caffeine. For some people, just stopping caffeine intake is all they need to do to stop their incontinence. A trial without caffeine for at least 3 weeks will indicate if caffeine is a factor in the loss of bladder control. Artificial sweeteners, such as Nutrasweet, may also be implicated in the loss of urine control.

Constipation

Constipation refers to infrequent, hard bowel movements that are difficult to pass. Severe constipation, which results in large amounts of stool remaining in the rectum, or outlet for the bowel, can decrease urine control by putting pressure on the bladder and urethra. People with constipation need to establish a regular bowel program before attempting to treat their urinary incontinence. Chapter 11 gives a detailed explanation of measures for preventing constipation.

Estrogen Loss

After menopause (change of life) the tissues of the vagina and urethra lose tone and moisture, as was mentioned in the previous chapter. This loss of tone can decrease the ability of the urethra to close tightly to prevent leakage. Sometimes, using an estrogen supplement can restore the tissue sufficiently to increase urine control. Not all women should use estrogen. If you suspect estrogen loss may be a factor in your urinary incontinence, check with your health care professional to discuss the problem and treatment options.

Persistent Incontinence

Sometimes people develop a loss of urine control that is not related to an acute problem or new treatment. *Persistent incontinence* is lasting and does not resolve after an illness is over or after adjustments of medications, fluids, or other measures for acute incontinence. Four types of persistent incontinence have been identified: overflow, stress, urge, and functional. The chart on page 19 lists characteristics for each type of persistent incontinence.

Overflow Incontinence

Overflow incontinence results when the bladder does not empty completely, either because of some form of blockage or because of poor bladder contraction. As more urine is made and sent to the bladder, it causes the contents to fill up and "overflow." Symptoms of overflow incontinence are (a) frequent dribbles in small amounts, (b) difficulty starting urination, (c) decreased force in the stream of urine, (d) stopping and starting while one is trying to empty the bladder, and (e) a feeling of not emptying the bladder completely.

Two mechanisms can cause overflow incontinence. One is caused by a blockage of the outlet tube to the bladder,

Signs of Persistent Incontinence

Overflow	Difficulty starting stream Interruption of stream Decreased force of stream Terminal dribbling Sensation of incomplete emptying
Stress	Loss of small spurts of urine with cough, sneeze, standing Loss of urine after physical activity, heavy lifting Often dry at night
Urge	Loss of urine after strong urge to void Loss of urine during sleep Usually loss of large amounts of urine
Functional	Physical, mental, or environmental limitations: Inaccessible toilet Poor lighting Difficulty removing clothing Physical disabilities, decreased mobility Dementia Psychological factors

or urethra, which can be due to an enlarged prostate gland, a tumor, or a narrowing of the urethra itself (see the illustration on page 20). The blockage allows only small amounts of urine out of the bladder at a time.

A second mechanism of overflow incontinence is poor nerve innervation of the bladder muscle, resulting in

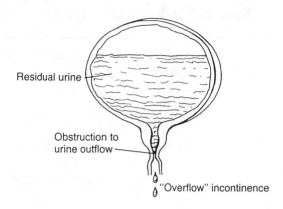

Residual urine

Obstruction to
urine outflow

"Overflow" incontinence

Blockage of urethra in overflow incontinence. (From *Nursing for Continence,* **1990, by K. Jeter, N. Fuller, and C. Norton, Philadelphia, W. B. Saunders. Reprinted with permission.)**

poor contraction of the muscle and, thus, less ability to empty the bladder. Some diseases that can affect nerve innervation in this way are diabetes, multiple sclerosis, and spinal cord injuries.

Overflow incontinence can be dangerous, because when the bladder does not empty completely urine can be backed up the ureters into the kidneys and cause significant damage to the kidney itself. If you suspect this type of urinary incontinence, a physician or nurse should be consulted.

Stress Incontinence

Normally when pressure rises in the bladder (as when a person coughs, sneezes, stands, or jumps) the outlet to the bladder, including the muscles along the urethra, is strong enough to override the pressure and keep urine from leaking. With stress incontinence the outlet is unable to counteract rising bladder pressure, resulting in leakage of urine. The majority of causes for stress incontinence are attributed to weakened pelvic muscles.

The pelvic muscles are a large band of muscles that form a sling to support the pelvic organs (the uterus and vagina, bladder and urethra, and colon and rectum). Various conditions can weaken these muscles,decreasing their ability to shut off the stream of urine. For women, pregnancy and vaginal delivery can damage the pelvic muscle group. During a vaginal delivery the vagina stretches from a diameter of 1 inch to about 4 inches to accommodate the delivery of the child. The movement of the baby down the birth canal (vagina), along with the force exerted by strong uterine contractions, causes stretching and possibly tearing of the pelvic muscles. The amount of damage relates to the size of the baby and the number of subsequent pregnancies and deliveries.

Obesity, or being overweight, also contributes to stress incontinence by weakening the pelvic muscles. Excess weight places pressure on the pelvic muscles. Many women have found that with weight loss stress incontinence improves. If you are overweight, you may want to discuss weight reduction with your health care professional as part of your treatment plan.

Weakness to the pelvic muscles can result in drooping or sagging of the pelvic organs. The bladder can drop down and bulge into the vagina. This is called a cystocele. Similarly, a rectocele can develop, where the rectum bulges up into the vagina. When a cystocele occurs, the bladder loses its normal position with the urethra. The normal angle where the bladder connects to the urethra is a natural mechanism to help shut off any urine leakage when abdominal pressure increases. This area is called the "bladder neck," and sometimes a surgical procedure to restore the bladder to its normal position will also restore bladder control.

Another factor in the ability of the urethra to seal off the bladder is the level of estrogen in the body. As women age and go through menopause there is a decrease in estrogen production in the body. A total hysterectomy, which can include removal of the ovaries, can also produce a sharp decline in estrogen production. As mentioned in Chapter 1, less estrogen results in changes in the vaginal and urethral tissue that lessen the ability of the muscle to maintain a tight seal.

Pelvic surgery can also result in stress incontinence. A hysterectomy (removal of the uterus), for example, can change the alignment of the bladder to the urethra, although many surgeons now try to account for this.

Stress incontinence can also occur in men, although this is uncommon. Men may experience leakage of urine with a cough, sneeze, laugh, or lifting following surgery on the prostate gland because of damage to the urethral outlet. Recovery usually occurs within 3 months after the surgery. If incontinence persists, reevaluation of bladder function should be pursued.

Urge Incontinence

Urge incontinence is often described as the inability to get to the toilet on time after sensing the urge to urinate.

Generally, urine loss is in large amounts, and often individuals need to urinate frequently during the night. The cause of this problem is not completely clear, but there appears to be a hyperactivity of the bladder muscle. The individual is unable to stop the muscle once it has begun to contract and empty the bladder. Some diseases that affect the nerves that transmit delay signals to the bladder are thought to be factors in the development of urge incontinence, such as multiple sclerosis, Parkinson's disease, strokes, or dementia.

Aging can make an individual more prone to develop urge incontinence because the bladder is less resilient and holds less urine than before. Local irritants, such as urinary tract infections or the pressure from constipation, can cause a temporary urge incontinence. However, in many cases, a definitive cause cannot be determined. Chapter 5 reviews treatments for urge incontinence and ways to relearn the ability to control the bladder muscle contraction.

Functional Incontinence

Some people have problems with urinary leakage even when the bladder and its associated structures are all working correctly. This is called functional incontinence and refers to other physical, mental, or environmental limitations that inhibit a person from toileting successfully. Physical handicaps such as arthritis or decreased ability to walk can make it difficult for a person to get to the bathroom in time to prevent urine loss. Some people depend on others to get to the bathroom and may not have such assistance available at the right time.

Individuals with cognitive impairment, or dementia, can develop a functional incontinence for multiple reasons. They lose the ability to recognize the body's signals of a full bladder, they may forget where the toilet is, or once they are there, they may forget how to use it. Additionally, people with dementia often have poor fluid intake. They may have severe constipation or any of the other acute causes of incontinence. They may have urge incontinence. One cannot assume that the incontinence is due solely to the dementia. Incontinence, along with dementia, is one of the leading factors in nursing home placement for individuals, because urine loss places a significant stress on caregivers. It is important that people with dementia who are incontinent receive a thorough evaluation and treatment program.

Environmental factors can also inhibit timely toileting. Some examples are poor lighting for finding the toilet at night, cluttered walkways, a bathroom door too small for a wheelchair, and a bathroom located too far from the bedroom or up a flight of stairs. Sometimes people refuse to toilet appropriately in order to meet a psychological need, for example, getting assistance by being helped with changing wet clothing. Several suggestions for managing functional incontinence are given in Chapters 6 and 7.

Mixed Incontinence

Unfortunately, the type of incontinence for a particular individual is not always clear-cut. In many cases more than one mechanism is at work and possibly both acute and persistent factors. A common problem is the person who has difficulty delaying the urge to void and also has urine loss with coughing or sneezing. Another person with a physical disability, such as arthritis, might have urge incontinence that is compounded by difficulty removing clothing in time to toilet appropriately. A physician or nurse who specializes in incontinence can help sort out contributing factors in incontinence. However, you can also follow some basic guidelines to increase your understanding of your particular problem with bladder control.

Evaluating Symptoms

The first thing to do when evaluating a bladder control problem is to review possible causes of acute incontinence and eliminate any that may be contributing to your urinary leakage. If you haven't already done this, review the first part of this chapter and follow any suggestions, such as stopping caffeine or increasing fluid intake.

Once acute causes of incontinence have been eliminated as much as possible, use the following symptom chart to identify the type of urine loss you have. Go down the chart and answer each question in the space provided. Then look at the symptom chart key. It will help you decide if your symptoms are suggestive of stress, urge, overflow, or functional incontinence. You will also be able to tell if your symptoms are suggestive of more than one type of incontinence. Once you have narrowed down what type of incontinence you may have, you can look at subsequent chapters in this book for initial treatment strategies.

Urinary Incontinence
Symptom Chart

	YES	NO
1. I lose urine when I cough.	___	___
2. I lose urine when I sneeze.	___	___
3. I lose urine when I laugh	___	___
4. I lose urine when I lift objects.	___	___
5. My urine loss is small amounts.	___	___
6. My urine loss occurs mostly during the day	___	___
7. I get a strong urge to urinate,then can't get to the toilet on time.	___	___
8. My urine loss is in moderate to large amounts.	___	___
9. I lose urine while asleep	___	___
10. I get up at night to urinate.	___	___
11. I have trouble starting to urinate.	___	___
12. My urine stream starts and stops during urination.	___	___
13. I have frequent dribbling.	___	___

Symptom Chart Key

If you answered "yes" to numbers 1–6, you may have stress incontinence. Refer to Chapter 4 for treatments.

If you answered "yes" to numbers 7–10, you may have urge incontinence. Refer to Chapter 5 for treatments.

If you answered "yes" to numbers 11–13, you may have overflow incontinence. Consult your health care provider.

Summary

Symptoms do not always exactly reflect the type of mechanism at work in urinary incontinence, but they can serve as treatment guidelines. The best person to evaluate urine loss is your health care provider. Chapter 3 will provide information about aspects of an incontinence evaluation and the health care professionals available to assist you.

Chapter 3

Seeking Professional Help

❖❖❖❖❖❖❖❖❖❖❖❖❖❖❖❖❖❖❖❖❖❖❖

Incontinence Care Providers

There are many health care professionals who can assist an individual who has urinary incontinence. The first place to start in seeking out help is your physician. Your physician may choose to perform the entire incontinence work-up, or only part of the evaluation, referring you to a specialist for further testing. Several health care professionals provide incontinence care, including urologists, gynecologists, nurse incontinence specialists, and geriatricians.

Urologist

A urologist is a physician who provides evaluation and treatment for disorders of the urinary tract in men and women, and disorders of the reproductive system in men. Urologists evaluate urinary incontinence through urodynamic testing, which measures bladder and urethral pressures, and cystoscopy, which allows them to look inside the bladder and urethra. Once the cause of incontinence is determined, urologists will prescribe treatment, which may include medications or surgery. A person can be referred to a urologist by the primary physician, or can seek out a urology evaluation on one's own. Check with your insurance carrier before an appointment to clarify if a referral is necessary.

Gynecologist

Gynecologists are physicians who specialize in the evaluation and treatment of the reproductive and urinary systems of women. Some gynecologists are also trained in urodynamic and cystoscopic testing. They provide a full range of medication and surgical treatments for urinary incontinence. If you are considering seeing a gynecologist for problems with incontinence, ask in advance about what services they offer.

Nurse Incontinence Specialist

Nurse incontinence specialists may have a clinical background in a variety of areas, for example, urology, gynecology, women's health, geriatrics, or enterostomal therapy. In general, nurse incontinence specialists provide a complete incontinence evaluation. Some, however, may only do a partial evaluation, with subsequent referral to a specialist for more in depth testing. Nurses provide a full range of incontinence management, but refer to specialists if surgical intervention is warranted or if the incontinence is not responding to treatment.

Geriatrician

A geriatrician is a physican who specializes in the treatment of older adults. Because incontinence is such a prevalent problem for adults over 65, many geriatricians are knowledgable about the causes and treatments for incontinence and can provide patients with either a complete or partial evaluation.

Elements of an Incontinence Evaluation

History

Regardless of the provider you see, there is basic information you will need to provide during an incontinence evaluation. The evaluation usually begins with a history, or a review of factors that might contribute to urine loss. Some providers will mail you a history form to complete prior to your first appointment. If not, you can use the following questions to organize your thoughts. Review them and write down your answers. Take your responses with you when you go for your initial incontinence evaluation. It will also be helpful for you to complete the symptom chart in Chapter 2.

1. When did the incontinence start? Did the leakage begin gradually or suddenly? Did anything bring it on (e.g., medication change, illness)?

2. How often do you lose urine (day/night)?

3. Is the amount of urine loss large or small?

4. How frequently do you urinate during the day and during the night?

5. What causes you to lose urine?

6. What present or past health problems do you have (e.g., diabetes, Parkinson's disease, frequent urinary infections)?

7. What are your current medications (prescription and nonprescription)? It would be best to take all medication with you to your evaluation.

8. How much fluid do you drink during the day?

9. How many caffeinated beverages do you drink in a day (e.g., coffee, tea, cocoa, soda)?

10. How many alcoholic beverages do you drink in day?

11. Do you have any problems with constipation or involuntary loss of stool?

12. Do you ever experience burning with urination or blood in the urine?

During the history interview, the health care provider may ask additional questions about your mood and about your eating, sleeping, and sexual habits. The health care provider may review your ability to perform daily self-care, such as getting in and out of chairs, dressing, and getting to the bathroom, to determine if functional ability contributes to the incontinence. The health care provider may also test your memory. If you have someone who helps with your daily functions, the health care provider may benefit from speaking with that person as well to get any additional information about your incontinence.

For many people, it is very difficult to talk about their problems with bladder control. If you have taken the time to ensure that you are seeing a health care provider who has expertise in the evaluation and management of incontinence, it should be worth the effort to share this personal part of your life, because urinary incontinence can respond very favorably to treatment. If after the first visit you do not feel the health care provider has a good understanding of your problem, or if you feel the person does not share your concern for your loss of bladder control, seek another health care professional to assist you.

Physical Examination

After the incontinence history is reviewed, your health care provider will perform a physical examination that is focused on elements that affect the urinary system. This often includes a brief evaluation of the neurological system, the abdomen, the perineum and vagina for women, the prostate for men, and the rectum.

Neurological Examination

The neurological examination is done to look for problems with the nervous system that can affect the function of the bladder. These problems are more common with illnesses such as diabetes, Parkinson's disease, strokes, and dementia. Your health care provider will evaluate reflexes, muscle strength, and your ability to differentiate sensations (sharp and dull).

Abdominal Examination

During the abdominal (belly) examination, the health care provider may listen over the abdomen with a stethoscope to hear the bowel sounds that indicate the intestine is working properly. The health care provider will also be looking for bladder enlargement or for a mass in the abdomen that could be putting pressure on the bladder (such as an intestine full of stool). This is done by pressing or feeling with the hand over the patient's abdomen. Let the health care provider know if you feel any discomfort during the exam, especially over the bladder area. This may indicate a bladder infection or an enlarged bladder.

Uroflowmetry. Some health care providers will want your bladder to be full for the abdominal examination. It is important that you not empty your bladder before your appointment. At some point you will be given a chance to urinate. You may be asked to void into a measuring hat that can be placed in the toilet or into a special toilet called a uroflow chair. This procedure, called uroflowmetry, measures the force of the urine stream, as well as the amount of urine. It provides additional information about the function of the bladder and the amount of urine your bladder can hold. You may also be asked to give a urine specimen at this time.

Pelvic Examination

A pelvic examination is an important part of the evaluation for women. The health care provider will be looking for the presence of a cystocele (see the illustration on page 36), rectocele (see the illustration on page 37), or dropping down of the uterus or vaginal walls. All of these suggest weakening of the pelvic muscles. It may be necessary to insert a speculum into the vagina to better visualize these changes in the pelvic organs, as well as to note any signs of infection or generalized inflammation of the vaginal walls or any other abnormalities that might contribute to incontinence. After the speculum is removed, the health care provider will insert one or two fingers into the vagina to better assess the size and placement of the pelvic organs. You may be asked to squeeze your perineal muscles around the examining finger, so the provider can evaluate the strength and tone of those muscles.

Rectal Examination

In both men and women, sensation around the anus may be checked, and a rectal exam will be done to evaluate the strength and tone of the anal sphincter. The health

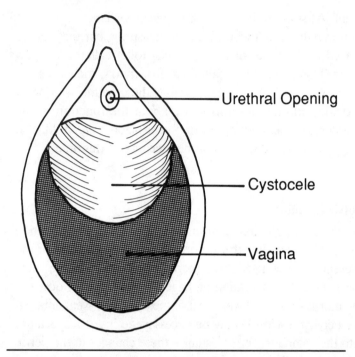

Weakened pelvic muscle with cystocele formation.

care provider will insert a finger into the rectum. Again, you may be asked to squeeze the muscles around the examining finger. In men, health care providers will also check the prostate gland for size and tenderness.

Stress Maneuvers

During the physical examination, and also during some of the diagnostic tests, you may be asked to do stress maneuvers. These include such things as coughing, bearing down as though having a bowel movement, bounc-

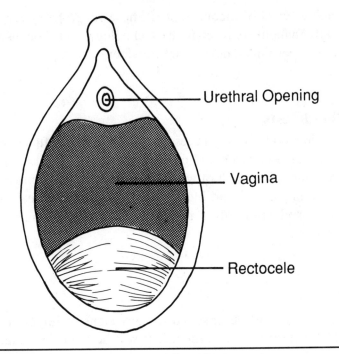

Weakened pelvic muscle with rectocele formation.

ing on your heels, or bending over. Leakage of urine during these activities is suggestive of stress incontinence. You don't need to feel embarassed if you have urine leakage; this is just what your provider needs to see in order to be confident of how best to help you.

Diagnostic Tests

In addition to a history and focused physical examination, certain tests help health care providers to diagnose specific types of incontinence. These range from very simple maneuvers to complex technology, and their use varies according to health care provider.

Blood Tests

Certain blood tests are necessary to check kidney function (blood urea nitrogen and creatinine), calcium levels, and blood sugar levels, all of which can affect bladder control. A rise in calcium and blood sugar can cause increased urine production, often resulting in frequent urination and leakage.

Urine Tests

Your urine will be checked for any signs of infection, which can cause incontinence. It will be important that you collect as clean a specimen as possible to be sure that bacteria that is normally on the skin does not get into the urine. You should be provided with a cup and towelettes. Open both first. Next, if you are female, separate the labia, or folds that cover the urethra, with your thumb and index finger. If you are male and uncircumcized, pull back the foreskin. Keep the labia or foreskin pulled back throughout the collection. Next, take a towelette and wipe the exposed area with a front to back motion (female) or inner to outer circular motion (male). Once the area is well cleaned, begin urination. Without stopping the stream, catch some urine in the cup. Remove the cup and finish urination.

After you have given the sample to your health care provider, he or she will have the urine examined under a microscope to look for signs of infection, such as the presence of white blood cells, bacteria, and red blood cells. If you have a urinary tract infection, you will need to take an antibiotic. For some people, infection may be the cause of urinary leakage, and once the infection is treated continence is restored.

If your health care provider sees red blood cells in the urine without other signs of infection, you may be asked to repeat the test. Blood in the urine is called hematuria. It may be caused by infection or menstruation, but it can also signify a serious illness that warrants further evaluation and should never be taken lightly. Women should tell their health care provider if they are menstruating at the time of the urine test.

Post-void Residual

After you have given your urine sample, the health care provider may briefly reexamine your abdomen. The bladder will then be checked for how much urine is remaining. This is termed the post-void residual. Normally, small amounts of urine may remain in the bladder after voiding, but larger amounts indicate the bladder is not emptying completely. Incomplete emptying may be caused from the bladder contracting poorly or from a blockage at the bladder outlet. Large postvoid residuals cause overflow incontinence and generally require further testing to determine what is inhibiting complete bladder emptying.

Bladder Ultrasound

Some providers use a small ultrasound machine to check postvoid residual. A gel is put on the abdomen, and an instrument is moved across the abdomen above the bladder along two angles. In less than 5 minutes the instrument is able to visualize the bladder and calculate the volume of urine remaining in the bladder.

Bladder Catheterization

More commonly, health care providers need to perform a bladder catheterization to determine post-void residual. While you are lying on the examination table, the area around the urethra will be cleaned with a bacteriocidal solution. Then a small sterile catheter will be passed through the urethra into the bladder (see the illustration on page 41). You may feel a little discomfort initially, but this should not be painful. When the catheter enters the bladder, any urine remaining in the bladder will drain out through the catheter and into a collection container where it can be measured.

Urodynamic Testing

Urodynamics are special diagnostic tests that measure how well the bladder, urethra, and pelvic muscles are functioning. There are several different types of urodynamic tests. The most common of these is cystometry (also called CMG or cystometrogram). Cystometry measures the pressure in the bladder as it is filled with sterile water and emptied. During cystometry, sterile water is instilled into the bladder through a small catheter. How the bladder responds to filling is recorded on a graph with

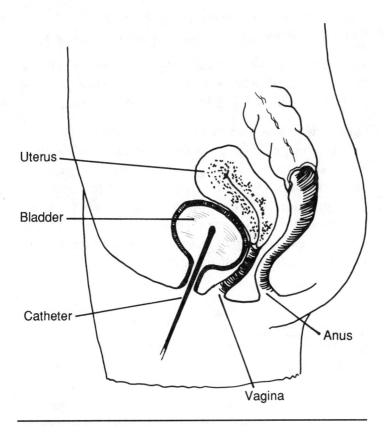

Insertion of catheter into the urethra.

special equipment. With this procedure the health care provider gets much information about bladder function: (a) the level of fluid in the bladder at which you get the first urge to void, (b) maximal bladder capacity, (c) the presence of bladder contractions that can't be controlled, and (d) any leakage with stress maneuvers. Immediately after the procedure, you will be asked to empty your bladder. This amount will be measured to give another indication of the ability of your bladder to empty completely.

Some health care providers do "simple cystometry" without the use of specialized equipment. They still can see how the bladder responds to filling, but do not have the visual graph.

Other urodynamic tests that require specialized equipment (manometry, pelvic floor electromyography, urethral pressure profilometry, voiding cystourethrography, cystocopy) can be performed to further identify other factors contributing to urine loss. Which additional test is needed is different for each individual. If any of these tests are recommended, ask your health care provider to explain the procedure so you have a better understanding of its purpose.

Voiding Record

An important piece of information can be a voiding record. This record describes from a day-to-day basis your normal voiding pattern and leakage episodes, along with associated activities and fluid intake. If a voiding record is requested, you will be given a form such as the one in Chapter 5. You may want to keep the voiding record in this book for 3 days and take that information with you to your appointment.

Summary

Many health care providers are gaining expertise in evaluating and treating urinary incontinence. As stated earlier, a good place to start in seeking help is your physician. You should be aware, however, that there are other professionals who could offer you assistance in incontinence evaluation and management. Choose a health care provider who understands and shows interest in evaluating and treating problems with bladder control. Be prepared for your initial appointment by taking with you your responses to the history questions and the symptom chart. Also bring all medications, both prescription and over-the-counter, that you are currently taking. If possible, take along a 3-day voiding diary. Try to make sure that your bladder is full for your appointment. If you have any questions or concerns about the incontinence evaluation, be sure to discuss these with your health care provider. Write down the questions as you think of them to be sure you recall them at your appointment. Together you and your health care provider can develop a plan of care to eliminate or significantly improve your urine loss.

Chapter 4

Regaining Control with Stress Incontinence

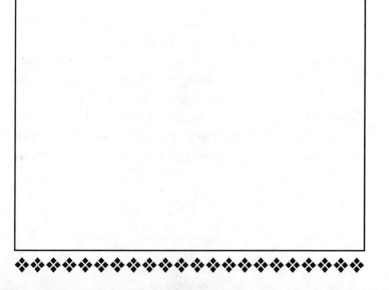

Pure stress incontinence is one type of incontinence that has shown good improvement with surgical intervention. However, recent research also indicates that less invasive treatments can also be very successful. Current recommendations are that in general, other treatments should be tried before surgery is considered. This chapter will review current nonsurgical treatments. The choice of treatment will vary depending upon the specific factors contributing to the loss of bladder control. Often positive results occur in the first few weeks, but a treatment should be given a trial of at least 3 months before it is considered a failure and another form of treatment is tried.

Weight Loss

Being overweight adds pressure on the bladder and the perineal muscles, thereby increasing the work of the bladder outlet in order to remain closed.

Losing weight, however, is never a simple, one-time task. It often requires a total lifestyle adjustment so that calories expended exceed calories consumed. If you need to address issues of weight loss, it is best to consult your health care provider for an appropriate exercise regimen and information on a healthy weight loss diet. You may benefit from consultation with a dietitian or involvement in a recognized weight loss program, where you can obtain the needed support for making a permanent lifestyle change.

Estrogen Replacement

Often stress incontinence is closely related to the tissue changes in the urethra after menopause, as has been described in Chapter 2. In addition to urinary incontinence, some women experience burning, vaginal dryness, or significant discomfort with intercourse due to the deficiency in the hormone, estrogen. For many women, replacing the estrogen lost after menopause is sufficient to stop urinary incontinence and may help resolve other menopausal symptoms as well. Estrogen replacement therapy (ERT) is also useful for women who are at risk for osteoporosis.

Estrogen Tablets

There are several regimens available for ERT. The most widely used is estrogen in a tablet form. If a woman has had her uterus removed (hysterectomy), estrogen alone is sufficient. However, if a woman still has her uterus, progesterone is taken with the estrogen to decrease build-up of the uterine lining, thus minimizing any risk of uterine cancer. The estrogen tablet is typically taken on days 1–25 of the month. The progesterone is generally given along with the estrogen on days 16–25 of the cycle, and many women experience harmless vaginal bleeding, or menstruation, during the days off both hormones. This menstruation generally does not cause cramps. Newer regimens of hormonal therapy are being studied to diminish the unwanted side effect of monthly menstruation. Some women on ERT also experience breast tenderness. Reducing the estrogen dose has been helpful in decreasing the degree of breast discomfort.

Vaginal Estrogen Cream

Another method of estrogen replacement is to use a vaginal cream. The cream is applied into the vagina with an applicator that is similar to a tampon. It is applied nightly for 2 weeks, then gradually tapered off over a 6-week period. Eventually women only need to apply a small quantity two to three times a week to maintain good urethral tone.

As with all medications, there are risks and benefits to ERT. This therapy should not be used in individuals with a history of:

1. breast cancer,

2. blood clots,

3. estrogen-dependent tumors,

4. uterine cancer, and

5. undiagnosed vaginal bleeding.

Some studies suggest that taking estrogen may have some protective benefit against heart disease. When used properly, estrogen is a safe medicine and very beneficial in the treatment of incontinence. Your health care provider can help you evaluate whether this would be an appropriate treatment for you.

Perineal Exercises

Women have been doing perineal exercises since Dr. Kegel introduced them in the late 1940s. The purpose of the exercises is to improve the tone of the perineal muscles, thereby increasing support for the pelvic organs, including the bladder. Improved tone also helps the bladder outlet, or urethra, to remain closed inspite of increased pressure in the bladder. Perineal exercises are not only recommended for women. Men who have had prostate surgery, or who have stress or urge incontinence, may also benefit from improving perineal muscle tone.

The most important part of perineal exercises is being able to identify the muscle you are exercising and the motivation to stick to an exercise program. People have often done perineal exercises incorrectly because they are tightening the abdominal muscles and buttocks but not exercising the correct muscle.

Pubococcygeal Muscle

The pubococcygeal muscle (PC) is a large muscle that goes from the anus up to the pubic bone (see the illustration on page 50). The PC muscle is one of the muscles that form the perineal muscle group. The PC muscle is responsible for maintaining tone and support for the pelvic organs and is the muscle group which responds to perineal exercises. The PC muscle can be difficult for many women and men to locate. One way to identify the PC muscle is to sit on a toilet ready to void. Put your knees as far apart as possible. Begin the urine stream and then try to stop it. The muscle you feel working to stop the urine stream is the PC muscle. (Don't expect to be able to shut off the urine stream completely.)

Another way that women can identify the PC muscle is to insert two fingers into the vagina. Try to squeeze

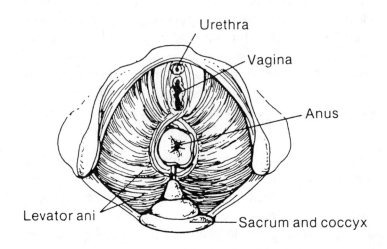

Pubococcygeal muscle. (From *Nursing for Continence*, 1990, by K. Jeter, N. Fuller, and C. Norton, Philadelphia, W. B. Saunders. Reprinted with permisssion.)

around these two fingers. Again, you should feel the muscle working. This method can also be a good way for you to check if the muscle tone is improving with the exercises.

A third method of identifying the correct muscle to exercise is to squeeze your rectum (anus). The sensation is similar to trying to stop from passing gas. For men, squeezing the rectum together, or trying to lift the base of the penis will help them locate the PC muscle. If you cannot identify the muscle at all, you may want to see a health care provider to help you.

Perineal Muscle (PC) Exercise Program

Once you have identified the PC muscle, you are ready to begin the exercises. Tighten the muscle, squeezing and pulling it inward, and hold it for 4 seconds. Then relax it for 4 seconds. This makes one exercise. Repeat the exercise 10 times. If the muscle seems to tire, drop back to only 5 exercises, or whatever level doesn't tire the muscle.

After 2 weeks, increase the length that you hold the tightened muscle to 6 seconds. You should always relax the muscle for the same amount of time. After another 2 weeks, increase the time to 8 seconds. By the end of 6 weeks, you should be able to contract the muscle for 10 seconds, which is the maximum amount of contraction time for the exercise.

We are currently recommending the exercise regimen described by Burgio and Pearce in the book, *Staying Dry*. Perineal exercises should be repeated three times a day, in different positions each time, either standing, lying, or sitting. Different positions are helpful because the muscle works a little differently in each position. Standing while doing the exercise is also important, because leakage is likely to occur in this position.

An example of the exercise program is:

1. Before getting up in the morning, lie in bed and do 10 exercises.

2. In the afternoon, while sitting in a chair, do another 10 exercises.

3. In the evening, when you are standing (perhaps during meal preparation), do another 10 exercises.

It is not necessary for you to do *all* three positions at the same time, but rather space the exercises out during the day so you do not fatigue the muscle.

In the beginning, set aside specific times when you will do the exercises and nothing else. This will help you to concentrate solely on the tightening and relaxing of the PC muscle. Once you become comfortable isolating the muscle, you can begin to do the exercise with other activities. Sometimes it is helpful to keep a record of exercises done.

It is important that you not expect results immediately. Some people do find improvement in the first few weeks. But most people need of few months of daily exercise to begin to note any benefits. If after a 3-month trial of the exercises you *don't* see any change, you should consult a health care provider for further treatment options.

Medications

In addition to estrogen, there are medications that work directly on the muscle along the urethra. These medications enhance the ability of the muscle to contract, thereby more effectively closing off the outlet to the bladder. Medications used to tighten the urethral sphincter are:

Generic Name	Trade Name®
Phenylpropanalamine	Dexatrim®, Ornade® Entex®
Pseudoephedrine	Sudafed® and others
Imipramine	Tofranil®

These medications have other uses as well. For example, some of these medications are contained in over-the-counter cold preparations, such as Sudafed®, which is a decongestant. Some of the medications used to tighten urethral tone can cause undesirable side effects such as an increase in blood pressure, rapid heart beat, and headache. In addition, Imipramine can cause a dry mouth and dizziness upon standing, which results from a drop in blood pressure. Imipramine has also been associated with falls in the elderly. Again, as with any medication, it is important to discuss with your health care provider the risks and benefits, as well as appropriate dosages, before using this treatment option.

Biofeedback

Many professionals who treat urinary incontinence are finding that biofeedback machines can help people better localize the perineal muscle and thereby improve the effectiveness of perineal exercises. Biofeedback is simply a way of giving input back to the person about the effectiveness of the muscle contraction. The degree of ability to shut off a stream of urine, or the pressure felt on fingers that are inserted into the vagina are two simple forms of biofeedback.

Biofeedback machines for urinary incontinence have some form of visual display that allows the person to directly see the perineal muscle contracting (see the illustration on page 54). Pressure measurements are obtained using various types of equipment. Some machines use a probe, inserted into the vagina or rectum, which directly

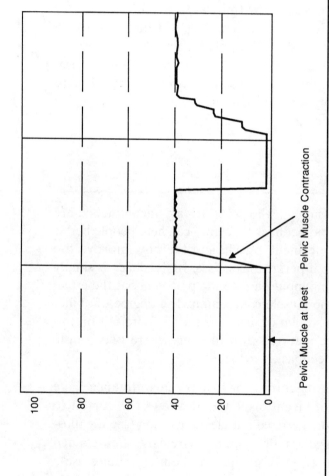

Pelvic Muscle at Rest   Pelvic Muscle Contraction

Visual display of perineal muscle contraction during biofeedback.

measures the pressure exerted during the perineal exercise (see the illustration below and on page 56). Others use electrodes placed around the anus that transmit the energy exerted when the muscle is contracted (see the illustration on page 57).

Many people have found biofeedback therapy to be a helpful tool for doing perineal exercises, especially those who have difficulty identifying the perineal muscle. Not all health care providers have this equipment, however. It is important to remember that while biofeedback is a helpful tool, it is not essential for learning perineal exer-

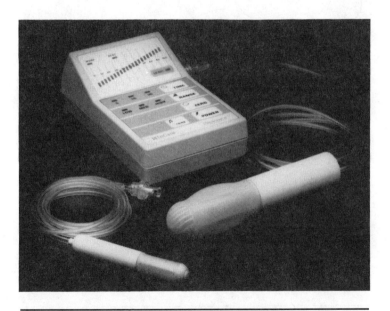

Vaginal and anal probes for biofeedback. (Courtesy of InCare Medical Products Division of Hollister Incorporated.)

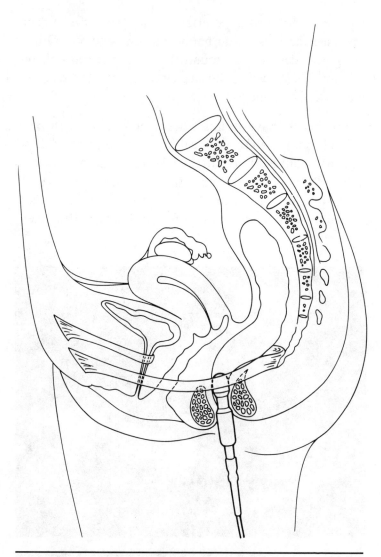

Biofeedback probe in place in the rectum. (Courtesy of InCare Medical Products Division of Hollister Incorporated.)

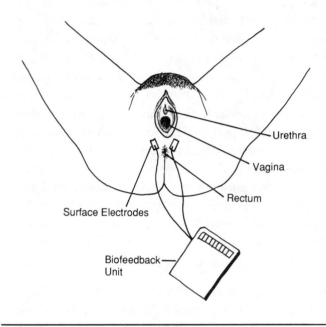

Surface electrodes for biofeedback.

cises. A skilled health care provider and motivation are the most important parts of any exercise program.

Perineal Stimulation

Another method available to increase perineal muscle tone is called electrical stimulation. Electrical stimulation has been beneficial for individuals who have a very weak perineal muscle, or who cannot voluntarily contract the muscle. The goal again is to increase the tone of the perineal muscle.

With this treatment, a probe similar to that used for bio-feedback is placed into the vagina or rectum and connected to a stimulating device (see the illustration on page 59). An electrical current is delivered from the stimulator to the probe and causes the perineal muscle to contract. The amount of electrical current needed is set by the health care professional in the clinic. The treatment is *not* painful. In general, people describe it as a pulling sensation in the pelvic area. When the electrical current is delivered, it causes the perineal muscle to contract. Voluntary contraction of the muscle along with the electrical stimulation will further enhance the effect of the treatment. The treatment is done for two 15-minute sessions a day for 6 to 8 weeks. Portable units allow people to do the therapy at home (see the illustration on page 60).

Although uncommon, incorrect use of the electrical stimulation can cause damage to the tissues of the rectum and vagina. Therefore, people who use the method need to be followed by their health care provider to assure proper use and to monitor progress.

Surgery

Several surgical procedures are available for women with stress incontinence. Women who have a moderate degree of stress incontinence and who have not benefited from a perineal exercise program may require surgery to alleviate the problem. The overall goal of a surgical procedure for stress incontinence is to restore proper positioning of the bladder and urethra, thereby restoring some of the

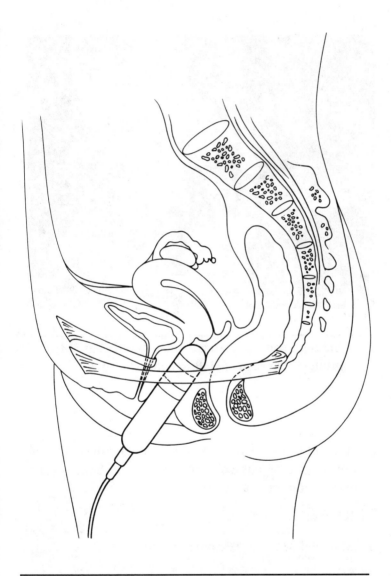

Electrical stimulation probe in place in the vagina. (Courtesy of InCare Medical Products Division of Hollister Incorporated.)

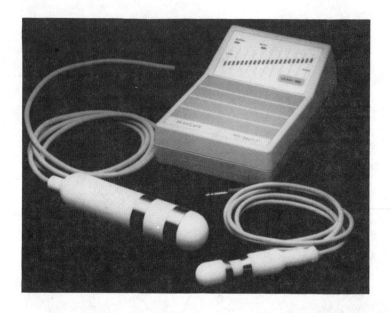

Portable electrical stimulator. (Courtesy of InCare Medical Products Division of Hollister Incorporated.)

natural mechanisms of stopping urine leakage. The surgical procedures used for stress incontinence require an incision either to the vaginal or abdominal areas. Several different types of surgical procedures exist. Some of the more common types are:

the Kelly procedure,

the Marshall-Marchetti-Krantz procedure, and

the Stamey procedure.

A vaginal sling procedure can also be performed for women who have severe damage to the perineal muscle.

A sling is created from muscle or from a synthetic material and inserted to help provide support to the urethra and to provide pressure to increase resistance and inhibit urine leakage.

Cure rates with surgical procedures vary from 50 to 95%. Both gynecologists and urologists are trained to perform surgery for stress incontinence and will best be able to evaluate your potential for benefit from a surgical repair.

Hysterectomy

For women who have been advised to have the uterus removed (hysterectomy), it will be important in many cases to also evaluate bladder function prior to surgery. Some women who experience weakening of the PC muscle and sagging of the uterus may actually not have a problem with urine loss because the sagging uterus is putting pressure on the urethra and keeping it closed. Once the uterus is removed in these cases, incontinence can develop. It is best to anticipate such problems so that the position of the bladder can be stabilized at the same time of the hysterectomy.

Prostate Surgery

Men who have had surgery of the prostate gland can sometimes experience stress incontinence due to damage to the sphincter. Perineal exercises can be helpful at reducing the incidence of stress incontinence in men who have undergone prostate surgery. Prior to surgery and 4 months after prostrate surgery, men should perform the perineal exercise program described earlier in this chapter.

Another treatment option for stress incontinence which can occur after prostate surgery is periurethral injections. Men who have had surgery to the prostate through the urethra can improve 80 to 85% with the use of a periurethral injection; however, only 50% of men who have had a radical prostatectomy, where the entire prostate gland and some surrounding tissue have been removed from an abdominal incision tend to benefit.

Artificial Sphincter

Men or women with total incontinence due to an incompetent sphincter can benefit from the placement of an artificial sphincter (see the illustrations on pages 63 & 64.) This involves the placement of a cuff around the urethra. The cuff is connected to a reservoir of water, usually placed in the abdomen, and then to a small bulb placed in the male scrotum or in the labial folds of a woman. The person can manipulate the bulb to fill the cuff with water to stop leakage, or drain the cuff to release the pressure on the urethra and allow the bladder to empty.

Periurethral Injections

Another procedure used for stress incontinence is called a periurethral injection. A periurethral injection involves injecting a polytetrafluorothylene material around the urethra, thereby adding pressure to help close the urethra. Approximately 75% of people with this procedure experience good to excellent results.

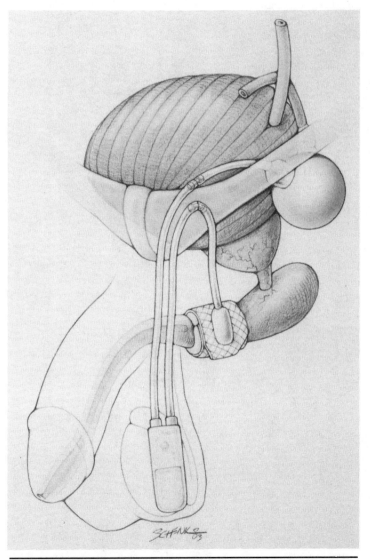

Artificial sphincter. (Courtesy of American Medical Systems, Inc., Minnetonka, Minnesota. Medical illustration by Michael Schenk.)

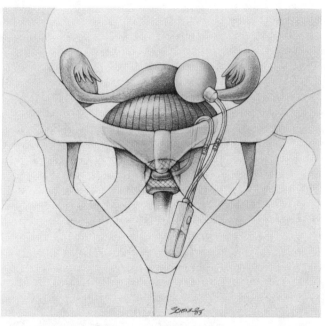

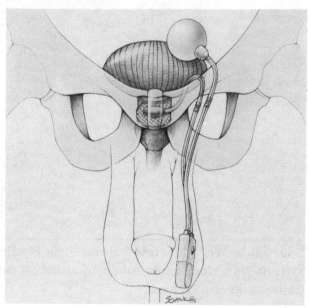

Penile Clamp

A penile clamp is a clamping device that is placed around the penis. When the clamp is closed it exerts pressure on the urethra causing it to close up and stop leakage (see the illustration below and on page 66). A penile clamp should be used with caution, as it can cause damage to the penis. Clamps must be fitted by a health care provider and generally are not the first management strategy tried. However, for select patients, a properly fitted clamp and good patient education can restore continence.

Summary

There are now a variety of treatments available to improve or cure stress incontinence. A person can safely begin with the accepted noninvasive treatments, such as

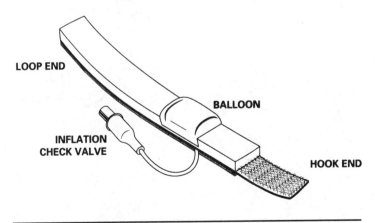

LOOP END

BALLOON

INFLATION CHECK VALVE

HOOK END

Penile clamp. (Courtesy of VPI, A Cook Group Company, Spencer, Indiana.)

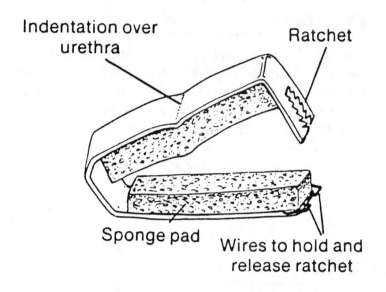

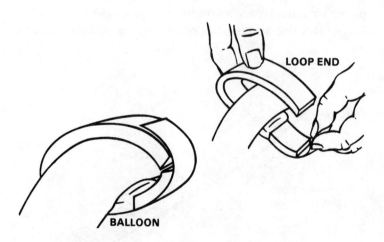

Penile clamp. (Courtesy of Cunningham Clamp Medical Marketing Group.)

perineal exercises, to see if improvement can be made. If perineal exercises alone are not successful, it would be important to pursue further evaluation and other treatment options with a health care professional who is trained in managing urinary incontinence.

Chapter 5

Regaining Control With Urge Incontinence

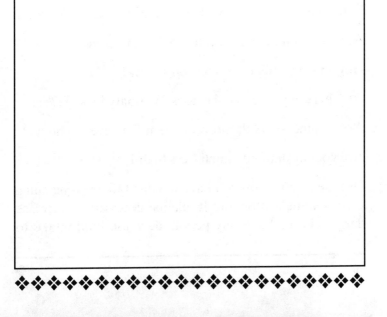

Many simple behavioral interventions have been shown to help urge incontinence. Surgery in all but rare cases will not help. It is important to first look at any temporary causes and treat them. Constipation, for example, can be a major factor in urge incontinence by placing additional pressure on the bladder. Constipation needs to be resolved before any treatment for incontinence will be effective.

Voiding Diary

A helpful tool is a voiding diary. For a 3-day period, record what time you void, how much you void (exact quantity is best, or else note "small" or "large"), any urine leakage, and factors contributing to urine leakage, such as coughing, sneezing, or standing up. Also record the amount, type, and time of all fluid intake. See the illustration on pages 71 and 72 for a sample voiding diary.

Once your diary is complete, review it for these elements:

Is fluid intake adequate (six to eight 8 ounce glasses per day)?

Are you drinking a lot a fluids before bedtime?

How much caffeine are you consuming?

Are there any associated causes to urinary leakage?

Are voiding intervals more frequent than every 3 hours?

Are voiding amounts small (less than 1 cup)?

Use the information you have obtained to begin planning your treatment program. It may be necessary to increase daily fluid intake. Many people decrease fluid intake to avoid the problems of leakage that occur with a full bladder. Ironically, this decrease in fluid intake may actually make the problem worse. The urine becomes more concentrated and serves as an irritant to the bladder muscle, stimulating more uncontrollable contractions. People with excessive fluid intake may need to see their health care provider to determine why they drink so much. Excessive thirst can be a symptom of diabetes or kidney problems.

Some people may need to try a 3-week period without caffeine. Limiting fluid intake after 6:00 p.m. may prove helpful if nighttime incontinence is a problem. Yet for others, decreasing the amount of fluid consumed may help limit urinary leakage. Urinary frequency, however, could indicate a urinary tract infection, and this should be checked out with your health care provider.

In general, an adult will void eight times or less in a 24-hour period. Small, frequent voidings are often the result of the worry that persons who are incontinent can develop. To avoid the embarrassment and discomfort of urinary leakage, a person with urge incontinence tends to go to the bathroom more frequently to prevent the bladder from getting too full. In the long run, however, this prevention strategy actually makes the problem worse, because decreased stretching of the bladder muscles decreases bladder function. It is essential to retrain the bladder muscle, with the goal of being able to go 3 to 4 hours between voidings.

Bladder Retraining

Persons with urge incontinence will often say, "When I gotta go, I gotta go." This statement indicates that the

DAILY VOIDING RECORD

TIME	AMOUNT VOIDED	LEAKING EPISODE? L = LARGE S = SMALL
12–1 AM		
1–2 AM		
2-3 AM		
3–4 AM		
4–5 AM		
5–6 AM		
6–7 AM		
7–8 AM		
8–9 AM		
9–10 AM		
10–11 AM		
11–12 NOON		
12–1 PM		
1–2 PM		
2–3 PM		
3–4 PM		
4–5 PM		
5–6 PM		
6–7 PM		
7–8 PM		
8–9 PM		
9–10 PM		
10–11 PM		
11–12 PM		

Voiding diary.

DATE: ————————

ACTIVITY AT TIME OF LEAKAGE	URGE PRESENT? Y OR N	AMOUNT/TYPE OF FLUID INTAKE

Voiding diary (continued)

bladder is in control instead of the individual. This is *not true*. Immediate voiding in response to an urge to void is not necessary. In fact, the urge sensation is mostly a message to you that the bladder is filling.

The purpose of bladder retraining is to help the individual reestablish control over bladder function. Before bladder retraining begins, and during the course of treatment, persons are instructed to keep a voiding diary. From the voiding diary, the health care provider can assess the individual's normal pattern of voiding and associated factors which may precipitate leakage of urine. In addition, the diary offers a method of monitoring the success of a bladder retraining program, both for the individual and the provider.

Scheduled Voiding

There are two common methods of bladder retraining: scheduled voiding and delayed voiding. *Scheduled voiding* works on fixed intervals of voiding, with a gradual increase in those intervals. Let's say an individual's voiding diary shows frequent voiding intervals of 1½ hours, with leakage occurring at each void. With scheduled voiding, this individual might be instructed to empty the bladder the first thing upon rising in the morning, and then every hour, on the hour, whether the person felt the urge to urinate or not, until going to bed at night. The person should not void in between times. The only exception would be to prevent a lengthened time between voidings that might occur during a planned activity, such as a show, church, dinner, or a wedding. In such cases void prior to the activity and reset the schedule accordingly.

Once the individual can maintain the initial schedule without many episodes of urine leakage, the schedule is increased by 30 minutes. Thus, in this example, the individual would increase the voiding interval to every 1½ hours. The goal of scheduled voiding is to gradually increase the time interval between voidings until achieving urination every 3 to 4 hours. It should be noted that as time intervals progress beyond 2 hours, setting an alarm to remind the person to urinate may be helpful in maintaining the program.

Delayed Voiding

Delayed voiding is another method of bladder retraining that helps increase the interval between voidings. Again, the person's normal voiding pattern is assessed, along with episodes of leakage. Instead of a set voiding schedule, however, the individual is instructed that every time the urge to void is felt, that urge should be delayed for 15 minutes. It's important that you empty the bladder at the end of the 15 minutes, however, and don't put it off, for a subsequent sensation of urge will probably be even stronger and harder to control.

Progress with delayed voiding is monitored by the use of a voiding diary. Once the individual is comfortable with the 15 minute delay, the length of time to delay the urge is increased by 15 minutes; in other words, the individual would wait 30 minutes after experiencing the urge to void before going to the bathroom and emptying the bladder. This timing sequence would progress until the goal of voiding every 3 to 4 hours is achieved.

In the beginning stages of bladder retraining, it is normal to experience a few accidents. This should not be interpreted as a failure. It takes time and practice to reestablish control over the bladder.

Controlling the Urge

There are several techniques that are beneficial to help a person get through an urge to void. The sensation of urge is nothing more than a feeling. The urge feeling comes in waves and can be quite intense. One technique to stopping the urge is to do three quick perineal muscle exercises, with no rest in between. Squeezing the perineal muscle sends a message to the bladder to stop contracting. As the bladder stops contracting and relaxes, the urge subsides.

A second technique to getting through an urge to void is to stop what you are doing, stay put, or sit down if possible. Try to keep the abdomen relaxed. When you are quiet and calm, it is easier to control the urge.

Many individuals with urge incontinence have an overwhelming desire to rush to the toilet in an effort to "beat the bladder" before emptying begins. Rushing, however, is the *worst* thing to do because it results in increased pressure on the bladder, along with movement of the bladder, that both increase the sensation of urge as well as stimulate the bladder to contract and empty. Rushing also interferes with the ability to concentrate on controlling bladder function.

For an individual with urge incontinence, the worst time to go to the bathroom is when the urge to void is at its peak. The best time to urinate is before the urge wave begins, or after the wave has successfully been eliminated or substantially reduced.

A third technique to assist with bladder retraining is doing activities that will distract the mind. These may include:

• balancing your checkbook,

• counting backwards from 100 by 7s,

• watching television,

• reading a book, or

• doing a craft.

The objective is to *not* focus on the bladder. Even using simple meditation techniques, such as imagining yourself somewhere else, can be helpful.

Remember, an urge to void is *not* a command, but merely a warning signal that the bladder is filling. Bladder retraining is an effective treatment for urge incontinence. With bladder retraining, the bladder capacity is increased, voiding intervals are lengthened, and the individual establishes control over the bladder, rather than allowing the bladder to control the individual.

Habit Training

Some people will not be able to follow a bladder retraining program because of mental impairment or lack of total control over bladder emptying. These people will benefit from a habit training program to prevent incontinence episodes. Two basic methods of habit training are fixed and patterned.

Fixed Habit Training

Fixed habit training refers to a set schedule for voiding. Often this is a schedule of going to the bathroom every 2 hours. It may include voiding prior to outings or other activities where access to bathroom facilities may be limited. This method of preventing urinary incontinence can be effective, but should not be used unless bladder retraining programs are not appropriate, because a fixed schedule will decrease the opportunity for the bladder to fill completely. Limited expansion of the bladder wall will further limit the ability of the bladder to respond to increased filling.

Patterned Voiding

Patterned voiding refers to scheduling toileting according to one's individual pattern of voiding. People do not usually use the bathroom on a fixed schedule. A voiding diary can help one determine what times are frequently used for voiding, and what times are more likely to have associated incontinence. The individual can then anticipate the need to void by going to the bathroom in the 30 minutes prior to the normal voiding time. The bladder is emptied before the sensation of urge develops, thereby preventing the leakage that also occurs with the urge.

Medications

There are several medications available that decrease the activity of the bladder muscle and improve the ability of the bladder to store urine. The most common class of drugs used to treat urge incontinence are called anticholinergics. Some examples are:

Generic Name	TradeName
oxybutinin	Ditropan®
propantheline	Pro-Banthine®

Another form of medication used to treat urge incontinence are drugs that possess both a milder anticholinergic function and a bladder relaxant property. Some examples are:

Generic Name	Trade Name
dicyclomine	Bentyl®
flavoxate	Urispas®

In addition, medications such as calcium channel-blocking agents (Verapamil®, Nifedipine®, and Diltiazem®), which are used to control blood pressure and heart rate, are thought to have some effect on bladder relaxation. This classification of drug, however, is not considered standard therapy for urge incontinence in this country, but may warrant a trial if a person has both elevated blood pressure and urge incontinence.

As with any medications, anticholinergics do have side effects. Persons taking these drugs may experience dry mouth, constipation, blurred vision, dizziness, confusion,

heart burn, and rapid heart beat. In addition, anticholinergics can also cause the bladder to relax too much, producing urinary retention (inability to empty the bladder).
In general, however, when used properly, these medications are safe. Studies have shown that more than half of
the people who have used anticholinergics for urge
incontinence experience benefit.

Health care providers may also place post-menopausal
women with urge incontinence on estrogen. Estrogens
may help strengthen the muscles around the urethra. For
more information on estrogen treatment and effects, refer
to Chapter 4.

All medications have potential to cause undesirable side
effects. Bladder training alone can cure urge incontinence
in many people. Therefore, for many individuals with urge
incontinence, perineal exercises and bladder training programs are initial treatments. If you're having difficulty getting the bladder to respond to a training program, however,
a small amount of medication may be all you need to begin
to see some results. Consult your health care provider.

Perineal Exercises

Although perineal exercises do not affect the bladder
muscle itself, they have a role in the treatment of urge
incontinence. For one, they increase the ability of the
bladder outlet to resist the increasing pressure caused by
the hyperactivity of the bladder muscle. Also, there is
some suggestion that they may help to override the urge
stimulus to empty the bladder. Thus they can be a useful

adjunct to bladder retraining methods. Refer to Chapter 4 for a complete description of these exercises.

Perineal Stimulation

The electrical current used in perineal stimulation has also been found to decrease hyperactivity of the bladder muscle. Again, refer to Chapter 4 for more information on this method for controlling urge incontinence.

Mixed Incontinence

We seem to get more complex as we age, and incontinence problems are no exception. Often people over 55 years old develop a mixed form of incontinence, with both stress and urge components present. The treatment, however, is similar. We usually recommend that people begin with perineal exercises and later add a bladder retraining program. Using an estrogen cream may be helpful. There are also medications that *both* delay action of the bladder muscle and enhance the outlet muscle. Surgery may help the stress incontinence, but don't expect a complete cure, because the urge incontinence will remain.

Summary

Persons with urge incontinence do not have to be a slave to their bladders. Many individuals have been cured or had their leaking episodes significantly reduced with the treatment options discussed in this chapter. If you think you have urge incontinence, keep a voiding diary for 3 days and try to evaluate what things might be affecting your loss of control. Consider one of the bladder retraining methods that have been outlined. Discuss treatment options with your health care provider. If your provider is not knowledgeable in the treatment of urinary incontinence, ask who you should be referred to for assistance, or seek out help on your own.

Chapter 6

Managing Functional Urinary Incontinence

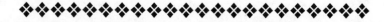

As mentioned in Chapter 2, individuals may have a normal functioning urinary tract and still experience urinary leakage due to an inability or unwillingness to toilet in a timely manner. This is termed functional incontinence.

Maintaining dryness or continence not only depends on the bladder's ability to store and empty properly, but also on an individual's dexterity, gait, sight, and cognitive (mental) function. Persons with arthritis or Parkinson's disease, for instance, may have difficulty getting out of a chair and walking down a hallway. Once the person reaches the toilet, he or she still needs to unfasten clothing and transfer onto the toilet safely. These simple processes, which we all take for granted, may take a considerable amount of time and effort for someone with mobility problems or other disabilities. Leakage of urine may occur because the person has limitations with walking, transferring out of a chair, and/or manual dexterity.

Persons with dementia (Alzheimer's disease) or declining mental function have also been classified as having functional incontinence although this may not always be the most appropriate label. As the dementia progresses, the person may need to be reminded to go to the bathroom, need visual cues to find the bathroom, be unable to recognize the sensation that the bladder is filling and needs to empty, or are unable to prevent a full bladder from emptying. More information about managing urinary incontinence in persons with dementia is discussed in Chapter 7.

To plan an effective treatment program for someone with functional urinary incontinence, several factors need to be evaluated. The individual not only needs to have an incontinence evaluation as described in Chapter 3, but also needs to have an evaluation of his or her functional status.

This chapter will present information on what a functional evaluation consists of and home adaptations to improve toileting skills. In addition, after you read this section, it is hoped that you will feel your situation is not hopeless. Much can be done to alter the home environment and clothing so toileting can be done in a timely and safe manner.

Functional Assessment

A functional assessment is quite simply an evaluation of a person's ability or inability to perform daily tasks such as bathing, dressing, transferring one-self onto or off a chair, walking, stair climbing, maintaining personal hygiene, managing bowel and bladder, and eating. Ideally the functional assessment should be performed in the person's home, but in most cases the initial evaluation is done in a clinic. There are several different health care providers who may perform a functional assessment. In most clinics, a physician or nurse conducts the functional assessment. Sometimes the person may be referred to an occupational or physical therapist for a functional assessment. During a functional assessment the health care provider will ask about or observe the person performing specific tasks (see the chart on page 86). The person or caregiver will also be asked how much time and assistance is required for the person to perform these skills.

Standardized Functional Assessment

Task	*Expectation*
Eating	The person can feed him/herself when food is placed within reach
Moving on and off a bed or chair	The person is able to come to a sitting position on the side of the bed and stand.
Providing personal hygiene	The person can wash his/her face and hands, comb hair, brush teeth, and shave.
Toileting	The person is able to get on and off a toilet, handle clothing, and use toilet paper.
Bathing	The person is able to perform a complete sponge bath, tub bath, or shower.
Walking	The person can walk at least 50 yards without help.
Stair climbing	The person can go up and down the stairs safely.
Dressing and undressing	The person is able to put on and remove all clothing.
Continence of bowels	The person is able to control his/her bowels without leakage.
Continence of bladder	The person is able to control his/her bladder both day and night without leakage.

Adapted from the Barthel Self Care Index. (Mahoney, F. I., & Barthel, D. W. [1965]. Functional evaluation: The Barthel Index. *Maryland State Medical Journal, 14*, 61–65.)

Home Structure

In addition to a functional assessment, the health care provider may also ask about the physical layout of the home. Some important information to provide is listed below.

1. Bathroom location: Is the toilet on the main floor or the second floor?

    What is the distance from the main living area to the bathroom?

    Is the bathroom doorway wide enough to accommodate a wheelchair or walker?

    Are there grab bars present to help the person get on and off the toilet?

    Does the person have to use the sink edge to push on in order to get on and off the toilet?

2. Lighting: Are the light switches easily accessible for the bathroom and the hallway?

    Are the light bulbs bright enough to illuminate the hallway and bathroom areas?

3. Clutter: Is the home cluttered?

    Are there obstacles that the person must walk around when going to the bathroom?

    Are there throw rugs in the home that the person could trip on?

4. Furniture: Does the persons favorite chair sit low to the ground, or does the cushion sag making it difficult to rise?

       Does the chair or couch have arm rests?

       Is it difficult for the person to get out of bed?

The information the health care provider obtains from the functional assessment will help guide recommendations for maximizing the person's abilities so toileting can be achieved. Some of the recommendations may require adaptations to the home; others may require alterations in clothing, and others may address the need for a mobility device such as a cane or walker.

Home (Environmental) Adaptations

In most cases, making home adaptations will not require major remodeling. Rather, simple changes to the furniture, bathroom, and lighting can significantly improve a person's ability to perform everyday tasks such as maintaining toileting skills. For functional incontinence, home adaptations may be centered specifically around the bathroom area. Some suggestions are as follows.

Distance and Location of the Bathroom

The distance to and from the toilet needs to match the individual's tolerance for walking. In most cases, the distance should be no more than 30 feet from the major living area in the home. In other words, if the individual spends the majority of his or her time in the living room, then the bathroom needs to be within 30 feet from that room.

The bathroom should also be located on the same floor where the person spends most of his or her time. If, for example, the bathroom is located on the second floor of a home, and the person is usually on the first floor, each time the need to urinate occurs the person must climb a flight of stairs. If the person has difficulty walking, then stair climbing will take a considerable amount of time, and may be unsafe. By the time the bathroom is reached it may be too late and leakage will have occurred.

Toilet Substitutes

For distance and location concerns, use of a toilet substitute can remedy the problem easily. A toilet substitute is a portable piece of equipment that can substitute for a regular toilet. One of the most commonly used toilet substitutes is a commode. Commodes come in two styles: with wheels and stationary (see the illustration on page 90). A stationary commode is placed in one area and remains there, whereas a wheeled commode can be easily moved from one place to another. Armrests, footrests, seating, padding, backrests, height, and urine collection containers can be selected to meet the individual needs of the person using the device. A commode requires routine emptying and rinsing to avoid odor of feces and urine in the sleeping or living areas. Remember, if a person has difficulty getting on and off a regular toilet, he or she will also have problems transferring on and off a commode. Therefore, a person with strength and mobility problems should first receive an evaluation from a health care provider before a commode is purchased. The type of commode pur-

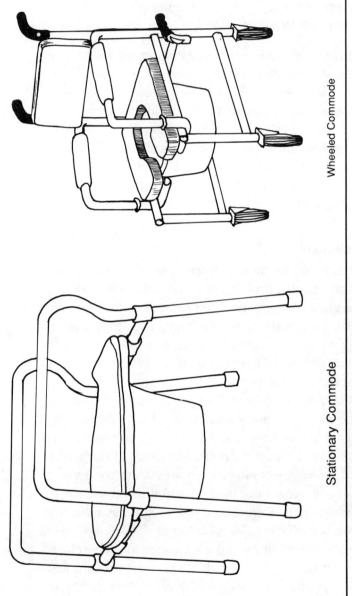

Stationary Commode

Wheeled Commode

Stationary commode and wheeled commodes.

chased should be one which offers the most security and stability for the person using it.

The need to use a commode may be difficult for the person and/or family to accept. If you feel you or someone you care for would benefit from a commode or any other home adaptation equipment, discuss these options with your health care provider. Your health care provider may refer you to a home health supply store, or to an occupational or physical therapist for equipment recommendations.

Urinals

Another type of toilet substitute is one that is hand held such as a urinal or bedpan. Urinals have been around for centuries, and only recently have their designs been improved. Urinals should be spill proof, easy to handle, empty, and clean (see the illustration on page 92). Most urinals will hold between 500–1,000 cubic centimeters of urine (which is between a quart to a gallon) and will have a handle or grip to hold onto during use.

Most commonly, urinals have been used for males. However, there are designs available for females and for those who are wheelchair bound. The design for females is slightly different from a standard male urinal. The opening is longer and wider to cup the urethra and funnel urine into a collection container (see the illustration on page 92). For persons who are wheelchair bound and wish to use a urinal, cushions can be designed with a cutout that can be removed so a urinal can easily be put in place.

Bedpans

Bedpans have also been used as toilet substitutes but are the least effective. Bedpans have a tendency to be poorly

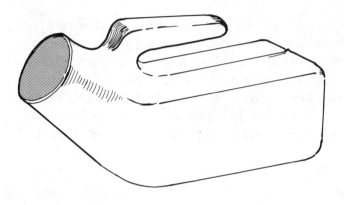

Male Urinal

Male urinal.

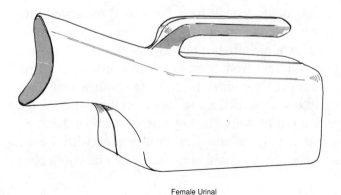

Female Urinal

Female urinal.

positioned, creating spillage and discomfort due to excessive pressure over the bony areas of the buttocks. In addition, for complete emptying of the bladder to occur, a person needs to be sitting at a 90° angle or almost upright. Due to the design of the bedpan, an upright position can be difficult to achieve. If a bedpan is used, then a fracture pan or "relaxed" adult pan is recommended because of the improved design (see the illustration below).

Transfer Aides

Transfer aides are devices that can assist persons with getting in and out of chairs or beds and on and off a toilet. For

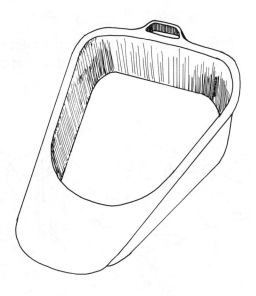

Relaxed bedpan.

individuals who have problems getting on and off a toilet, specially designed rails can be installed in the bathroom to improve the person's ability to toilet. If railings are recommended, they need to be properly installed. There are a variety of rails available. Some attach to the floor along either side of the toilet (see the illustration below). The most common type of railing used, however, are railings that attach to the wall (see the illustration on page 95). If a wall railing is recommended, the rail should be attached near the toilet, be well anchored, and have a depth of less than 2–3 inches from the wall to prevent slippage of one's hand or arm behind the rail. In addition, the rail needs to be placed at the correct angle and height for the person using it. In general, diagonal placement of a longer rail at the front of the toilet is most helpful (see the illustration on page 96). A good resource for rail installation would be your local home health or medical supply store.

Commercially available towel racks and sink edges are not designed to take the strain and stress that is applied

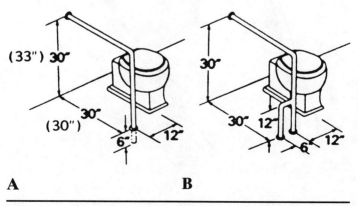

Floor-mounted rails. (Courtesy of the Bradley Company.)

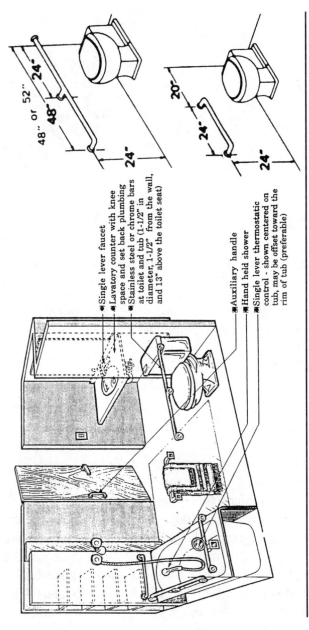

- Single lever faucet
- Lavatory counter with knee space and set back plumbing
- Stainless steel or chrome bars at toilet and tub (1-1/2" in diameter, 1-1/2" from the wall, and 13" above the toilet seat)

- Auxiliary handle
- Hand held shower
- Single lever thermostatic control - shown centered on tub, may be offset toward the rim of tub (preferable)

Wall-mounted rails. (Wheelchair accessible bathroom art courtesy of North Carolina Department of Insurance, Jim Long, Commissioner, and Jeff Kanner, Architect, Chief, Building Accessibility Section. Grab bar art courtesy of the Bradley Company.)

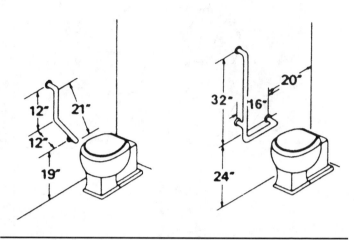

Diagonal rail. (Courtesy of the Bradley Company.)

repeatedly when the item is used as a transfer aide and, therefore, are not recommended for this use.

Raised toilet seats

To help with transferring, the toilet seat itself should be at a correct height. For most persons the seat should be 17–18 inches from the finished floor. If the toilet is lower than 17 inches, it does not have to be replaced with a higher model. A raised toilet seat can be purchased and secured onto the existing toilet, increasing the seat height and making it both easier and safer to get on and off the toilet (see the illustration on page 97). For some persons, however, once the toilet seat is at the correct height for transferring, they have difficulty moving their bowels or emptying their bladder. This may be due in part to losing the squatting position needed for good evacuation. Placing a footstool under the person's feet after he or she has gotten onto the toilet can be helpful.

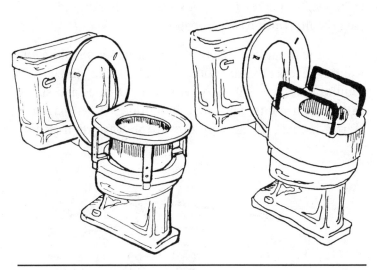

Raised toilet seat.

Clothing Adaptations

During a functional assessment a health care provider may find, or a family member may report, that the person with incontinence has difficulty managing his or her clothing. The problem may be that the hands are weak, or perhaps there is paralysis from a previous stroke. The simple task of using zippers and buttons then requires an increase in time or may be impossible to perform without assistance. Thus, leakage may occur even though the toilet is reached in time. Simple adaptations can be made to clothing to improve toileting skills.

For men, Velcro® fly closures are easier to open than a zipper. Altering the fly opening to extend down to the crotch seam makes for easier use of a hand held urinal (see the illustration on this page).

Women with limited function of their hands should avoid wearing layers of underclothing. Slips, girdles, and corsets require time and agility to get out of. Dresses and skirts, rather than pants, are more functional. A wraparound skirt is easiest for moving out of the way when getting

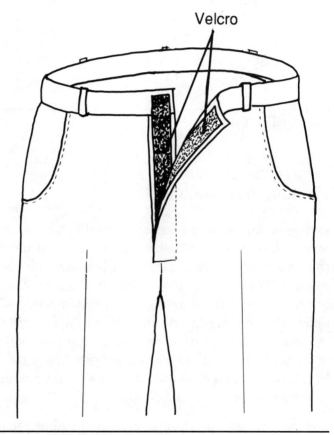

Velcro

Trouser adaptation for urinal use.

onto the toilet. If pants are worn, ones with elastic waist-bands, such as sweatpants, are preferable.

As with zippers, buttons can be replaced with Velcro® strips. Clothing items that open and close in the front are easier to remove than items that are secured in the back.

Walking Devices

Incontinence can also occur because a person may have difficulty with walking to the toilet. Difficulty with walking may be caused by problems with bones, muscles, joints, the nervous system, or environmental factors such as slippery floors, poor lighting, and poor footwear. Regardless of the cause, before purchasing a walking aide a thorough evaluation by a health professional should be performed. Once the evaluation is complete, the health care provider will have a better understanding of the cause of the walking problem and can recommend the most appropriate type of walking device. Many different types of mobility aides are available. Canes, walkers, crutches, and wheelchairs can significantly improve stability and speed of walking. Mobility devices need to be fit specifically to the person using it. Therefore, devices should be purchased from a credible medical or home health supply store, or from an occupational or physical therapy department.

Summary

Many simple alterations can be made in the home and with clothing to improve toileting skills for someone with functional incontinence. However, because of the large number of options available, and the numerous underlying causes for functional decline, environmental and functional assessments should first be performed by a health care provider. Only then can proper management be initiated and recommendations for the most appropriate equipment be made.

Chapter **7**

Dementia and Urinary Incontinence

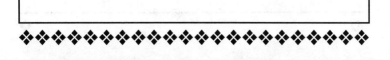

For most adults, cognitive function or the ability to perform intellectual tasks such as thinking, memory, perceiv-
ing, communicating, orienting, calculating, and problem
solving remains intact as they age. Dementing diseases,
the most common of which is Alzheimer's disease, repre-
sent a progressive decline in the ability to perform these
intellectual tasks. Alzheimer's disease occurs in 6% of
adults over 65, 10% aged 75–85, and 20% in persons over
85 years of age (Heckler, 1985). All too often caregivers/
family members and health care providers assume that
the onset of incontinence is just another aspect of dementia. Although urinary incontinence can coexist with
dementia, it is seldom an inevitable feature. Continence
(maintaining dryness) is so ingrained in most people that
it is often one of the last social skills to be lost in a person
suffering from dementia. For many persons with dementia
other causes of urine loss such as urinary tract infections,
constipation, diabetes, and prostate problems are often
overlooked and untreated. The urine loss experienced by
persons with dementia may also be caused from poor
functioning of the bladder and/or urethra, as seen with
stress and urge incontinence (see Chapters 4 and 5) and,
therefore, needs to be fully evaluated.

An incontinence evaluation for someone who has dementia should include not only an assessment of physical
causes as described in Chapter 3, but also an assessment of
cognitive or mental status. This chapter will provide information on components of a cognitive assessment and
strategies that can be used to decrease the episodes of urinary leakage for persons who have dementia and urinary incontinence.

Cognitive Assessment

An assessment of cognitive function can range from simple orientation to time, place, and person, to the ability to perform abstract reasoning and problem solving. Several different health care providers may perform a cognitive assessment. In most clinics a physician or nurse conducts a cognitive evaluation. Components of a typical mental status evaluation include testing of orientation, memory, attention, calculation, ability to name objects, ability to follow verbal and written commands, and ability to write a sentence and copy a drawing. A short version of a cognitive evaluation will be used in clinic settings and will take about 10–15 minutes. The chart on page 104 illustrates some typical questions that can be asked during a cognitive evaluation. From the brief cognitive evaluation the health care provider can discover if mental decline is present, what areas of intellectual function are affected, and decide if further testing is needed.

For persons who have dementia and incontinence, the forgetfulness that is characteristic of the disease may account for the person's inability to communicate his or her toileting needs. Below are some factors that may contribute to urinary incontinence in a person with dementia:

• Forgetting to toilet

• Loss of the ability to inhibit a bladder contraction

• Loss of the awareness of the need to void

• Forgetting where the toilet is located

- Being able to walk to the toilet or transfer on and off the toilet alone

- Difficulty getting dressed and undressed

Cognitive Examination

Area Testing	Questions
Orientation	What is the year, season, date, and month?
Memory	Given the name of three common objects to remember, and asked to recall those objects later on in the evaluation.
Attention/Calculation	Go backwards from 100 by 7s, or spell WORLD backwards.
Ability to name objects	Shown common objects and asked to name them.
Ability to follow verbal commands	Given a three-step command to perform.
Ability to follow written commands	Given a written sentence to read and follow.
Write a sentence	Asked to write a sentence. The sentence must contain a subject and a verb.
Copy a figure	Shown a figure and asked to copy it on a piece of paper.

From Folstein, M. F., Folstein, S., and McHugh, P. R. (1975) "Mini-Mental State: A Practical Method for Grading the Cognitive State of Patients for the Clinician." *Journal of Psychiatric Research, 12,* 189–198.

If you are providing care for someone with dementia who also has urinary incontinence, the first step toward treatment is to seek out a health care provider to perform a full incontinence and cognitive evaluation. Caution needs to be used to avoid the general assumption that urine loss is a natural progression of the dementing disease. If your health care provider does not feel adequately prepared to perform an incontinence and/or cognitive evaluation ask him or her to refer you to another professional. A geriatric clinic should have providers who could perform both evaluations.

Many strategies are available to help caregivers devise a program that will maximize functional and memory ability of the person with dementia. Some of the more commonly used strategies will be discussed next.

Urinary Incontinence Strategies to Assist the Person with Dementia

For persons with dementia, visual and verbal reminders (called "cues") can be very beneficial for maintaining toileting skills. This is especially true in the earlier stages of dementia when the person can still understand what these visual and verbal cues mean.

Visual Cues

In the early stages of dementia, the ability to indicate the need to void and to carry out the task of toileting is still present. As the disease progresses to the late stages, persons with dementia may forget where the bathroom is located, how to use buttons and zippers, or recognize the urge sensation. Visual and verbal cues to remind someone with dementia to go to the bathroom are extremely helpful.

Caregivers also need to be aware that for persons with dementia communication of personal and physical needs can occur through channels other than speech. Wandering, pacing, fidgeting with clothing, and general restlessness can be a signal of the need to void. Interpreting these signals and providing assistance with toileting or using visual cues as to the location of the bathroom can be helpful. Here are some examples of visual cues that other caregivers have found useful:

• Arrows or footprints painted or placed on the floor leading the way to the bathroom.

• Painting the bathroom door a bright contrasting color.

• A large picture of a toilet placed on the outside of the bathroom door.

• Posting a sign on the outside of the bathroom door that says toilet or bathroom.

• Using night-lights or leaving the bathroom light on at night.

Verbal Cues

Verbal cues are spoken reminders that can be used to help persons with dementia remember to perform a task such as toileting. Verbal cues for toileting need to be individualized. Some persons will understand "It's time to go to the bathroom." For others terms such as "pee," "pass water," or "go number one," are better understood. Once you find a term that is understood by the person, use that cue consistently to avoid confusion. Verbal cues can also be used with toileting programs to assist the person with dementia to maintain dryness.

Toileting Programs

Toileting programs are very effective at decreasing the number of wetting episodes and reestablishing the toilet as the appropriate place for urination. The success of a toileting program is dependent on the availability and motivation of the caregiver. One of the most popular toileting programs used with persons with dementia is called "scheduled toileting."

Scheduled Toileting

Scheduled toileting occurs at a set time interval. For example, if the schedule is set for every 2 hours, begin after the first morning void. If the person urinates at 7 a.m., then the next toileting will be at 9 a.m., then 11 a.m., and so on until bedtime. In general, a toileting program is not carried out during the night. However, some caregivers have found it helpful to toilet the person with dementia at least once during the night. If a nighttime program is desired, it should be individualized according to the needs of the person and caregiver.

Positive statements should always be offered when the person uses the toilet appropriately. Comments like,

"That's great that you stayed dry" or "It's wonderful that you urinated in the toilet" can improve the toileting program. In addition, spending social time with the incontinent person when he or she toilets correctly reinforces toileting behavior. Negative comments about wetting episodes should always be avoided. Remember the person with dementia is not wetting to get attention, or to irritate the caregiver.

Patterned Toileting

Another type of toileting program is called "patterned toileting." Patterned toileting takes into account the incontinent person's individual pattern of voiding. The person's voiding pattern is assessed by keeping a voiding diary for 3 days. Urine can be measured by having the person void into a plastic container or pail then pour the amount voided into a standard measuring cup. Many clinics have a special measuring container available called a toilet hat that can fit into any standard toilet. You may want to ask your health care provider if you can obtain one.

The diary will show if there is a consistent pattern to voiding and wetting episodes. Once the pattern has been established, the person is encouraged to void during the 30 minutes before the time when he or she would normally urinate or experience wetness. Following is an example of a patterned toileting diary.

According to the sample diary the person would be toileted at 6:30 a.m., 9:00 a.m., and 11:45 a.m.. The caregiver

Time	Amount Voided	Urine Loss (Small/Large)
7 a.m.	150 cubic centimeters	large
9 a.m.	none	no loss
9:30 a.m.	200 cubic centimeters	large
11:30 a.m.	none	no loss
12 noon	250 cubic centimeters	small

would continue to keep a diary to evaluate if the patterned schedule is sufficient in decreasing wetting episodes.

As stated earlier, toileting programs such as scheduled and patterned toileting are dependent on the availability and motivation of a caregiver. If you are a caregiver for someone who has dementia and you feel a toileting program would be beneficial, discuss this option with a health care provider. Together you can devise a program to meet the needs of all persons involved.

Summary

There are many treatment strategies available to help persons with dementia who may also have urinary incontinence. Persons with dementia can benefit from the use of simple visual and verbal cues and toileting programs.

The first step toward treatment, however, is a comprehensive evaluation. The evaluation of urinary incontinence for a person with dementia will not only include assessment of bladder function but will also include assessment of functional and cognitive (mental) ability. Successful programs can be developed but require creativity and patience for everyone involved: the person with incontinence, the caregiver, and the health care provider.

Chapter 8

Bowel Function in the Elderly

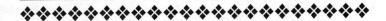

As persons age many factors make them more prone to develop difficulties with bowel function. This chapter includes a brief description of the normal working of the bowel, along with a discussion of what changes can occur with aging. Subsequent chapters will contain more de–tailed information about two specific bowel problems that can develop in the elderly.

Normal Bowel Function

Food and drink are processed in the body through the gastrointestinal tract, often referred to as the GI tract. It takes an average of 2 to 3 days for food to complete its transit through this system. The illustration on page 113 shows the various parts of the GI tract, which will be described below.

Upper GI Tract

Food is initially broken up by the teeth and moistened by saliva. The act of swallowing propels the food into the esophagus, a 12-inch, hollow, muscular tube connecting the mouth with the stomach. The combined actions of gravity and wave-like movements of the muscles of the esophagus advance the food downward toward the stomach. These wave-like movements are called "peristalsis" and occur throughout the GI tract. The sphincter (i.e., muscle) at the lower end of the esophagus opens to allow the food to pass into the stomach and then closes to prevent stomach con-tents from coming back up the esophagus.

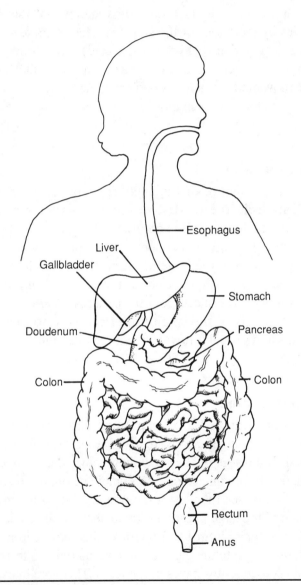

Gastrointestinal tract.

Once in the stomach, the food is broken down into smaller particles by secretions of the stomach. One of these secretions is a strong acid (hydrochloric acid). The stomach is composed of layers of muscle that also have wave-like, peristaltic movements which mix and grind the food. Small portions of the food are then moved into the small intestine.

Small Intestine

A primary function of the small intestine is to absorb nutrients from the food. The small intestine is coiled inside the abdomen and is approximately 20 feet long. It receives up to 8 quarts of food per day, but only about 1 quart passes on to the large intestine. The small intestine also mixes food with a variety of hormones, with mucus, and with digestive juices from the pancreas. Various muscle movements of the small bowel continue to mix the contents and propel it toward the large intestine.

Large Intestine

The large intestine is 4 to 5 feet in length and is the principal organ determining the consistency of stool, or feces, that is formed. It consists of the ascending colon, the transverse colon, the descending colon, the sigmoid colon, the rectum, and the anus (see the illustration on page 115). One major function of the large intestine is the reabsorption of salt and water. Anywhere from 1 to 2 quarts of fluid passes from the small intestine into the colon each day, and only up to 1 cup of fluid subsequently leaves in the feces. The large intestine also contains bacteria that break down the sugars and waste material remaining in the digested food.

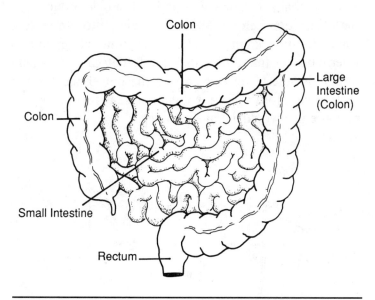

Large intestine.

Large intestine.

The large intestine also uses peristaltic movements to pass its contents toward the rectum at an average rate of a little over 2 inches an hour. Just taking in some food will stimulate these movements, but they also occur at periodic intervals. Stronger peristaltic waves occur spontaneously throughout the large intestine three or four times a day when the colon is filled. This is termed the gastrocolic reflex, and it often occurs following a meal. The muscle activity of the large bowel also mixes the contents.

Rectum and Anus
The final evacuation of bowel contents, or defecation, is a complex process involving the rectum, internal and

external anal sphincters, and perineal muscle groups (see the illustration below). Material moving into the rectum stimulates the rectum to contract. This contraction initiates a sensation of fullness, or the urge to defecate. A person usually is able to delay emptying the bowel because the rectum can hold a large volume without increasing the pressure that would initiate emptying.

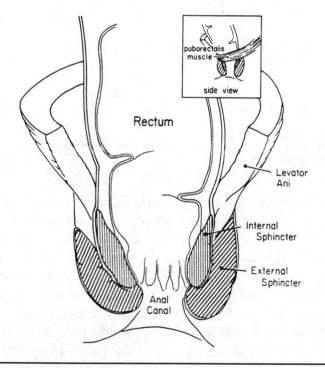

Rectum with anal sphincters and perineal muscles. From Stone, J. T. (1991). Managing Bowel Function. In W. C. Chenitz, J. T. Stone, & S. A. Salinburg (Eds.), *Clinical Gerontological Nursing* (pp. 214–232). Philadelphia: W. B. Saunders. Reprinted with permission.

The rectum has two bands of muscle called sphincters which help to control emptying. The internal anal sphincter normally maintains a level of contraction that keeps the anus closed. However, when the rectum fills with material, the internal anal sphincter relaxes, allowing the rectum to hold more contents. As the sphincter adjusts to the amount of material held in the rectum, it may regain some of its original tone and also help to keep the contents from emptying.

The external anal sphincter, which functions opposite the internal anal sphincter, tightens when the rectum fills, making sure that none of the contents are evacuated. As more material enters into the rectum, the external anal sphincter continues to contract or tighten, up to a maximum point. Beyond this point, the external anal sphincter is no longer able to tighten and may no longer stop defecation.

In addition to the anal sphincters, the puborectalis muscle is important for maintaining control over defecation. This muscle forms a sling around the rectum, creating an angle between the anus and the rectum (anorectal angle). This angle helps to stop the passage of stool (see the illustration on page 118). If the muscle is relaxed, causing the ano-rectal angle to increase to more than 110°, there is less ability to control the evacuation of material from the rectum.

Nerve Stimulation of the Bowel

The nervous system is important in bowel control. Nerve stimulation to the muscles of the bowel increases as the bowel fills with material. This stimulation coordinates the

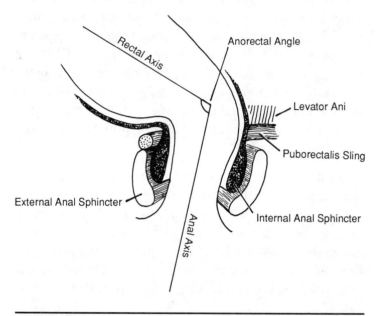

Anorectal angle.

muscle movements of the bowel that propel the contents toward the rectum.

There also is a center for defecation in the brain which allows voluntary control over the process. Nerve impulses from the brain can both stimulate and inhibit the movement of stool in the bowel, as well as the process of defecation itself. As with urinary control, this is a learned behavior in childhood. When one gets the stimulus from the rectum that filling has occurred, one can voluntarily send signals to stop evacuation. These signals then tell the rectum and the internal anal sphincter to continue to relax to receive more material. The signals also alert the puborectalis muscle and the external anal sphincter of the need to remain contracted and closed. If this signal to delay is not given, the contents of the bowel will be evacuated because the puborectalis muscle and the external anal sphincter also respond to local reflex stimulation, causing them to relax and allow the contents to pass.

Process of Defecation

The process of defecation occurs with the relaxation of the puborectalis muscle and the external anal sphincter, causing descent of the muscles and evacuation of bowel contents. Increased abdominal pressure by pushing down helps to empty the bowel, although the entire contents of the descending colon could be emptied by means of colonic contractions alone. Usually, however, only the contents of the rectum are cleared. Very small stools, such as those less than a $\frac{1}{2}$ inch in diameter, are difficult to evacuate because of the lack of stimulation of the rectal sensors.

Functional Factors

Bowel control also depends on the ability to recognize the signals from the rectum indicating the need to defecate, the ability to physically get to an appropriate place, as well as the ability to remove necessary clothing. These elements are the same as those described in Chapter 6 on functional urinary incontinence, and similar treatments would be applicable.

Factors in Normal Bowel Function

In summary, several factors are necessary to ensure normal bowel function. These include (a) the normal delivery of feces to the rectum, (b) the ability of the rectum to store the contents, (c) adequate functioning of the internal and external anal sphincters, (d) intact rectal and anal sensation, (e) an intact nervous system, (f) normal mental recognition of rectal signals, (g) the motivation/ability to make an appropriate response to the perceived need to defecate, and (h) adequate function of the puborectalis muscle (see the chart on page 121).

Changes with Age

Problems with bowel function are not automatic consequences of aging. However, several changes in the body with age can make one more prone to developing problems because they affect one or more of the factors described above that are necessary for normal bowel function.

Normal Aging Changes

Several processes occur throughout the body that ultimately have an impact on the function of the bowel. As

Factors Necessary For Normal Bowel Function

Normal passage of stool through the bowel

Adequate storage capability in the rectum

Proper functioning sphincters

Intact nervous system

Ability to perceive rectal fullness

Ability to respond appropriately to sensation of rectal fullness

Adequate function of puborectalis muscle

one ages, teeth can decay or be lost. If these are not replaced, food is not chewed properly to begin the process of digestion. A decline in the sensations of taste and thirst may affect the type of food and amount of fluid consumed, which will greatly affect the type of material handled by the bowel.

As one ages, the blood vessels can become somewhat hardened and develop a thicker lining which can reduce the blood supply to the bowel. This decreased blood supply can make the nerve stimulation and muscle movements less effective. This factor may explain why in some persons there seems to be a delay in the amount of time it takes for food to pass through the GI tract, which would increase the likelihood of hard, dry stool formation because of excess water removal.

Connective tissue changes, as such occur with thinning of skin and wrinkling, also occur in the GI tract and may decrease the flexibility and strength of the supportive structures. Less support reduces the resistance of the bowel to stress or increased pressure. There may be some loss of nerves stimulating the bowel, but, overall, little is known about changes in the nerves in the GI tract.

Changes within the Bowel

Several changes in bowel function occur with aging that affect one's ability to delay defecation. There is overall less pressure exerted by the internal and external anal sphincters, along with less response by the external anal sphincter to rectal filling. Therefore, less volume of stool would be needed to overcome the ability of the external anal sphincter to prevent defecation.

With aging there is a decrease in the ability of the rectum to continue to relax in response to increasing volume. Again, the need to defecate would come at a lower volume. Elderly individuals are also more likely to have decreased sensation of rectal fullness, resulting in less awareness of the need to defecate. Age-related changes in the spinal cord can decrease the nerve conduction to the anus, resulting in sphincter weakness and a predisposition to leakage of stool.

Lifestyle Factors

Lifelong habits can become accentuated as one ages and can have a significant impact on bowel function. Exercise is an important stimulant of muscle action in the bowel, and limited exercise promotes slower movement of food through the GI tract. Limited fluid intake, less than six to eight glasses or cups per day, decreases the amount of fluid entering the large bowel and can result in dryer, harder stools. Persistant use of laxatives can diminish the ability of the bowel to evacuate its contents without such assistance.

Disease-related Factors

Chronic diseases that often develop as individuals age increase the risk of bowel problems because these diseases can be debilitating, decreasing the potential for adequate exercise and possibly damaging specific parts of the bowel. Older adults also can require multiple medication regimens, often with side effects that include bowel problems. These factors will be further discussed in the following chapters.

Summary

It is important to recognize that despite these changes in the bowel that occur with aging, most individuals maintain adequate bowel control. The amount of function available in youth is generally well above that needed for minimum control, so even with some losses in the older adult, this minimum level can often be maintained. Being more aware of the mechanisms for bowel control and the elements that change as one ages will help establish good bowel habits that will prevent problems from developing, or perhaps diminish existing problems. The next two chapters will provide more detail about the separate issues of constipation and fecal incontinence, including specific measures for evaluating and treating these problems.

Chapter 9

Understanding Bowel Problems

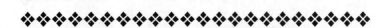

Two common bowel problems for older adults are constipation and fecal incontinence. Although they can be very different problems, they can also be interrelated. Both have a significant impact on the life of an individual, contributing to other health problems and potentially lowering self-image and the desire to socialize. The resultant isolation can cause further problems. Understanding the factors that contribute to constipation or fecal incontinence can help determine ways to prevent occurrence or to improve the situation. This chapter will provide information about the causes of constipation and fecal incontinence, as well as ways to determine which causes might be operating in a particular situation.

Constipation

The term "constipation" may have a variety of meanings. For the purposes of this book, we will define constipation as infrequent, difficult bowel movements. Some medical definitions say that less than three bowel movements in a week constitute constipation. Yet some people can have frequent movements, but they are in small, hard quantities that may also be considered constipation.

It is estimated that 2 to 7% of people over the age of 70 have constipation, which is similar to younger persons (Wald, 1990), although up to 30% may describe themselves as constipated (Whitehead, et al., 1989). Older persons, especially women, are more likely to use laxatives to maintain regularity.

Fecal Incontinence

Fecal incontinence is the involuntary leakage of bowel contents. The prevalence of this problem increases with age in both men and women. It is estimated to affect 3 to 4% of the elderly who live at home, 10 to 25% of hospitalized individuals, and up to 50% of those in nursing homes (Wald, 1990).

Multiple factors can contribute to the development of either constipation or fecal incontinence in the older individual, and often more than one factor is contributing to the problem. Many of these factors can be modified to improve or cure bowel problems, but it will be important to discuss these issues with a health care provider in order to sort out all of the potential causes and possible solutions.

Causes of Bowel Problems

Gastrointestinal Disease
Diseases of the bowel can affect an individual's ability to control evacuation. Cancers, inflammation of the bowel, infection, and trauma can all cause difficulty with bowel function. Some common gastrointestinal problems affecting bowel control are irritable bowel syndrome, diverticulosis, and diarrhea. Each problem responds to a different treatment, so it is important to be evaluated by your

health care provider to determine the cause and decide on the most appropriate treatment.

Irritable bowel syndrome can begin in young to middle-aged adults and is more common in women. Often people sense severe abdominal bloating and pain and an urgency to defecate, but are only able to expel a few small pellets. Variation in stool consistency may occur, ranging from constipation to diarrhea.

Diverticulosis refers to the development of abnormal herniations or sacs in the lining of the colon, usually from increased pressure within the colon. It is very common, especially in older persons, being present in 70% of people over 70. Diverticulosis often causes no problem for people, but sometimes the sacs can trap food residues and bacteria and become inflamed. This condition is called diverticulitis. It can be very painful and may require antibiotic therapy. Constipation is often an associated problem for people with diverticulosis.

Diarrhea is a common sign of gastrointestinal disease. Loose stools do not provide enough bulk to stimulate normal mechanisms for bowel control and are more likely to result in fecal incontinence. Diarrhea can be due to infection of the bowel with bacteria or parasites, sometimes occurring after antibiotic treatment. It can also develop with severe constipation, where only liquid stool is being passed. This cause is discussed in more detail in the section on fecal impaction.

Tarry, black-colored stools, may indicate bleeding in some part of the gastrointestinal tract. If you notice black stools, notify your health care provider.

Chronic Health Problems

As people get older, they are more likely to develop one or more chronic illnesses. Often these illnesses, or the medications used to treat these illnesses, can cause either constipation or fecal incontinence. Diseases that affect the nervous system can have a significant impact on bowel function by decreasing the nervous stimulation to the bowel. Examples are strokes, Alzheimer's disease, Parkinson's disease, or injuries to the spine. The result may be a slowing of the time it takes food to pass through the bowel, causing dryer, harder stools.

Moderate to severe mental impairment, as in Alzheimer's disease, can result in loss of the ability to stop the rectum from emptying once the sensation of filling occurs. The person still may sense the urge to evacuate the bowel, but is often unable to delay evacuation.

Mental decline can also reduce the ability of the person to remember how to respond to the urge to defecate. He or she may not remember where the toilet is, or know what to do when arriving there.

Another chronic health problem for some people is hypothyroidism, which develops when the body no longer makes enough thyroid hormone. It results in an overall slowing of the body's function, also slowing down the movement of food through the bowel and causing constipation. Conversely, too much thyroid hormone, hyperthyroidism, may result in diarrhea.

Medications

Older adults often take a number of medications for conditions such as high blood pressure, arthritis, and high cholesterol. Many of these medications can affect the function of the bowel. Pain medications, especially narcotics, can slow the motility of the bowel, resulting in constipation. Medicines for depression or for relaxing the bowel and bladder can also decrease motility. Diuretics can decrease the amount of fluid excreted in the bowel. Iron supplements often cause constipation. Antacids with aluminum hydroxide will promote constipation, whereas those with magnesium tend to cause diarrhea. Some heart and blood pressure medications can also contribute to constipation. Excessive replacement of thyroid hormone can result in diarrhea, as well as some antibiotics. The chart on page 131 lists common medications that can affect the bowel. It will be important to review both prescribed and over-the-counter medications that you use with your health care provider to see if any adjustments can be made to improve bowel function.

Diet

Fiber in foods can decrease constipation. Fiber is a food element that remains undigested as it moves through the stomache and small intestine and on into the large intestine. It increases the weight of stool, decreasing transit time through the gut and making the stool soft and easy to pass. More information about fiber intake is given in Chapter 11.

Foods that are high in fat content, as well as refined breads, can be very constipating. Drinking a large amount of tea is also thought to promote constipation.

Drinking insufficient liquids can increase hardness and dryness of the stool bulk. Older persons may not drink

Common Effects of Some Medications
on Bowel Function

Type	Constipation	Diarrhea
Narcotic pain medications	X	
Antidepressants	X	
Bowel and bladder relaxants	X	
Blood pressure medications	X	
Diuretics	X	
Iron	X	
Antacids	X	X
Thyroid hormone	X	X
Antibiotics		X

enough liquids because they normally have a decline in the awareness of thirst.

Bowel Habits

People often develop irregular patterns of evacuation, not always responding to the natural reflex to empty the bowel. Delayed evacuation will increase absorption of water from the bowel contents, making them hard and dry.

In our rushed society, people often don't take adequate time for evacuation of the bowel. They can be embarrassed about this normal bodily function. It's important to ensure privacy, adequate facilities, and sufficient time so that the bowel is emptied completely.

Lifestyle

A sedentary lifestyle can promote constipation because the limited physical activity can weaken the abdominal muscles that support the intestine. This slows down the passage of food through the bowel. Physical disabilities that limit activity will have a similar effect.

Laxative Abuse

Many older people overuse laxatives. A common belief in the early 1900s was that without a daily bowel movement, toxins would build up in the body. Many people still believe it is harmful if they do not empty the bowel daily and resort to laxative use to ensure this function. Persistent use of laxatives, however, can cause more problems over the long run because the bowel loses the ability to empty on its own. Types of laxatives and which ones may be safer to use will be discussed in Chapter 11.

Structural Causes

Fecal incontinence can develop when there is a change in the normal bowel structure that is necessary to control evacuation. Structure changes may be present at birth, or can occur with trauma or surgery. Childbirth, for example, can weaken the pelvic muscles, with resultant descent of the rectum and loss of the anorectal angle (see Chapter 8, the illustration on page 118). Repeated straining with defecation can also weaken the pelvic muscles. The loss of the anorectal angle will decrease the ability to delay defecation, and fecal incontinence will result.

Trauma, such as with childbirth, or repeated straining with defecation can also damage the pudendal nerve, a primary nerve for bowel function, by pressing it against the spine. Nerve damage eventually affects muscle control, with subsequent weakening of pelvic muscles and the external sphincter. A stretch injury may also result in nerve damage. Such damage can make it more difficult to stop the unwanted passage of stool, but it can also make it more difficult for a person to voluntarily evacuate a solid mass.

Chronic constipation and years of laxative use will also change the structure of the bowel. Excessive stretching may damage the nerves that stimulate evacuation. Also, the bowel wall may become thin and stretched and fail to respond to filling, resulting in less ability to tighten the external anal sphincter. Megarectum or megacolon can develop, which refers to an abnormal enlargement of the bowel size. All of these changes promote severe constipation, as well as making it more difficult to voluntarily empty the bowel.

Fecal Impaction

Fecal impaction is the blockage of the bowel by large amounts of stool. The solid mass of stool does not move well through the bowel. Only liquid or soft stool that can get around the impaction reaches the anal canal, resulting in evacuation that is much more difficult to control.

Fecal impaction can result when a person has long-standing problems with constipation, and it is the most common cause of fecal incontinence. Related factors are decreased activity, a diet low in residue, inadequate fluid intake, as well as certain medications.

Fecal impaction can be confusing for people because it frequently appears to be simple diarrhea. What is really underlying constipation looks like fecal incontinence. It is important to pursue the cause of persistent diarrhea before treating it with antidiarrheal medication, which would make an impaction significantly worse, possibly obstructing the bowel completely.

Environmental Factors

There are many factors apart from the structure and role of the bowel itself that contribute to the loss of bowel control. These factors include physical, mental, or environmental limitations that inhibit a person from toileting successfully. Examples are physical handicaps, facility access, adequate lighting, and the ability to recognize the appropriate toileting facility. Sometimes people develop problems with incontinence after they are hospitalized. This is usually a temporary problem that is related more to the change in environment, change in diet and fluid intake, change in mobility, and change in medications, rather than being related to any permanent change in bowel function. Chapter 6 extensively discusses various environmental factors of urinary incontinence that are also applicable to persons with fecal incontinence.

The timing of bowel evacuation is another important factor in maintaining adequate control. If a toilet is not accessible when the normal urge to defecate occurs or when a laxative takes effect, incontinence may result.

Psychosocial Concerns

Emotional and psychological factors also have an impact on the gastrointestinal tract. An emotional reaction to stress can alter bowel function, causing constipation or diarrhea. Depression can result in constipation through many factors: poor diet/fluid intake, lack of activity, or not responding to the sensation of fullness and thus delaying appropriate evacuation of the bowel.

Summary

Understanding possible causes of bowel problems sometimes helps people sort out simple things they can change to improve their own bowel function. The following chapter will review elements of a more in-depth evaluation by a health care provider.

Chapter 10

Evaluating Bowel Problems

Further evaluation with a physician or nurse can be helpful to get a more complete picture of causes and treatment options for constipation or fecal incontinence. You can start with your primary health care provider. If initial evaluation does not improve the problem, it may be necessary to seek the help of a specialist in gastroenterology.

History

A thorough evaluation of constipation or fecal incontinence begins with a complete history of the problem. Typical questions might be:

1. How long have you had the problem?

2. Was the onset sudden or gradual?

3. What was your normal pattern of bowel evacuation before developing constipation or incontinence?

4. What is the consistency of the stool (liquid, soft, hard, normal)?

5. Is there straining with defecation?

6. What are your toileting habits?

7. If you have fecal incontinence is it during the day? the night? both? Small or large amounts? Are there related factors such as inablity to get to/find toilet? inability to remove clothes? specific foods or medicines? a sense of urgency prior to incontinence? lack of warning? What have you done to improve the problem?

In addition, it will be important to review medications. This includes not only those prescribed by a doctor, but all the over-the-counter medications that are used. What kind of laxatives are used? Are enemas employed?

A diet history can be very helpful. Sometimes a person feels the diet contains sufficient fiber and fluids, but when intake is accurately recorded, will find deficiencies. Write down everything you eat and drink for a 3-day period, including approximate amounts, and take this with you to your appointment.

As mentioned before, other health problems are also important. These include any history of anorectal trauma, as in surgeries, difficult childbirths, or repeated straining at defecation. Other related factors might be nervous system injury, as with stroke, Parkinson's disease, dementia, back surgeries, radiation therapy, or the nervous system changes that can occur with diabetes. In addition, urinary incontinence, immobility, inflammatory bowel disease, problems with overall muscle function, and bowel infections should be noted. The chart on page 140 lists elements included in a history for bowel problems.

Bowel Record

A daily record of bowel movements can be very helpful in describing the problem and possible coexisting factors, especially in the case of fecal incontinence. The record should be kept for a few days and should include the time and consistency of bowel movements, including any episodes of incontinence. You should also note anything

Elements of a History for Bowel Problems

Onset of problem

Frequency of evacuation

Stool consistency

Toileting habits

Medications

Laxative use

Diet, fluid intake

Other health problems

Prior surgeries or trauma

Bowel record

you use to empty the colon, such as laxatives or enemas. Food and fluid intake are also important to record, for example, one cup of coffee, one tuna sandwich, half an apple, and one piece of chocolate cake. Physical activity can be noted, as well as anything else that seems to be associated with the loss of bowel control. This information will then provide some keys for treatment. A sample bowel record is shown in the illustration on pages 142–3.

Physical Examination

After reviewing the history and bowel record, your health care provider will perform a focused physical examination to evaluate some of the factors in bowel function. This often includes an examination of the abdomen, rectum, as well as the nervous system. A basic evaluation of the ability to perform daily activities and/or a simple test of mental ability may also be done if it appears these factors are contributing to the problem.

Abdominal Examination

The health care provider will listen with a stethoscope to the abdomen to hear the sounds made by the working of the bowel. The abdomen will also be felt to see if any stool is present in the bowel, or any other masses noted.

Rectal Exam

It will be important to inspect the area around the anus, both at rest and with bearing down, to see if there is significant descent or protrusion of the rectum through the anus. The skin is also inspected for any signs of irritation or breakdown and the existence of hemorroids. A gloved, lubricated finger is inserted into the anal canal to check for fecal impaction or rectal masses, as well as to ascertain the strength and control of the external anal sphincter. Some providers may use an anoscope, a small instrument that is inserted into the anus to allow visualization of the canal itself.

Nervous System

Your health care provider may check reflexes, muscle strength, and your ability to differentiate sharp and dull

DATE:_____

TIME	BOWEL		STOOL CONSISTENCY (hard, soft, fluid) & Amount (large, small)	USE OF SUPPOSITORY (number) or ENEMA
	Incontinent	Normal		
12-1 AM				
1-2 AM				
2-3 AM				
3-4 AM				
4-5 AM				
5-6 AM				
6-7 AM				
7-8 AM				
8-9 AM				
9-10 AM				
10-11 AM				
11-12 AM				
12-1 PM				
1-2 PM				
2-3 PM				
3-4 PM				
4-5 PM				
5-6 PM				
6-7 PM				
7-8 PM				
8-9 PM				
9-10 PM				
10-11 PM				
11-12 PM				

Bowel record.

URINE (amount)	FLUID INTAKE	FOOD INTAKE (poor, fair, good)	PHYSICAL ACTIVITY (none, poor, fair, good)
		Breakfast	
		Lunch	
		Dinner	

Bowel record (continued)

sensations in order to evaluate the nervous system. It will be important to check the reflexes and sensation around the anus to be sure that the sphincters are receiving normal nerve impulses.

Diagnostic Tests

Your health care provider can order some tests to further evaluate the bowel. It may be necessary to consult a specialist in gastroenterology for some of the testing. An abdominal x-ray may be taken to determine if the colon is full of stool.

Stool Tests

If diarrhea is part of the problem, a thorough workup may be warranted. This includes obtaining stool specimens to check for parasites or certain bacteria. A 72-hour stool collection may also be done to check for fat content, which can indicate absorption problems in the bowel.

Blood Tests

Blood tests may also be ordered to look for further causes of bowel problems. These might include blood cell counts, blood sugar, thyroid and calcium levels, kidney tests, and electrolytes.

Colonoscopy

Additional tests can help determine a cause for bowel problems. Proctosigmoidoscopy or a colonoscopy may be ordered. In these tests, a scope is inserted into the bowel to look for any growths or areas of inflammation. Medication to relax you and decrease discomfort is often given for the colonoscopy.

Sometimes a barium enema is done as a way to visualize the bowel. An enema is used to instill contrast medium into the bowel. The contrast is seen on an x-ray, revealing any obstructions or masses.

Specialized Testing

Often constipation or fecal incontinence can be treated with little testing, but sometimes the expertise of a specialist in gastroenterology is needed. Several tests of bowel function are available.

X-ray techniques are used to evaluate bowel structure. One test involves the injection of a small amount of barium into the rectum. A small metal chain is placed into the anal canal, allowing the x-ray to clarify the angle between the anal canal and the rectum. These tests give information on bowel capacity, the anorectal angle, and how much the pelvic muscles descend with defecation.

Manometry

Anorectal manometry is a test to measure various anal and rectal pressures, sensation, and the ability of the rectum to adapt to filling. One type of test is perfusion manometry, which uses a catheter placed in the anal canal, measuring pressures both at rest and with squeezing of the pelvic muscle. A second method is balloon manometry, which uses a three-balloon set-up. One balloon is placed at the external sphincter, one at the internal sphincter, and one into the rectum. As the balloon in the rectum is filled, the pressure responses of the internal and external sphincters are measured (see the illustration below). Normally, as the rectum fills, the internal anal sphincter relaxes, and the external anal sphincter tightens. Individuals receiving balloon manometry will be asked to have a bowel movement prior to the procedure. Sometimes a small enema is used to help complete evacuation.

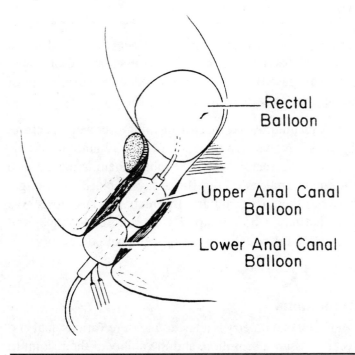

Balloon manometry. (From Schiller, L. R. [1986]. Fecal Incontinence. *Clinics in Gastroenterology, 15*[3], 687–704. Reprinted with permission.)

Electromyography

Electromyography is a test where electrodes are attached around the anus. This test measures nerve supply and muscle response, looking for any nerve or muscle problems that might cause fecal incontinence.

Continence Measures

There are also several tests to evaluate the ability to prevent leakage of bowel contents. In the test of continence for a solid sphere, a small sphere with an attached string is inserted into the anus and then the weight is measured that will pull the sphere through the sphincter. A similar test measures the ability of the individual to retain $1\frac{1}{2}$ liters of water instilled into the rectum.

Summary

The evaluation of bowel problems can be as simple as a basic history and as complex as anal diagnostic testing. The evaluation will determine what might be contributing to the problem and, therefore, what measures might make the situation better. The following chapters contain specific treatment measures for constipation and fecal incontinence.

Chapter 11

Managing Constipation

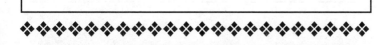

Constipation is not normal aging and has many treatment options. You may be able to sort out some basic causes in your own situation and make some initial adjustments that solve the problem. In many cases, however, it will be important to seek out the help of your health care provider to better understand contributing factors, to make sure health problems have been addressed, and to develop a plan for adequately managing these problems.

The management of constipation has typically focused on three main areas: diet and fluid intake, exercise, and toileting habits, as summarized in the chart below. In addition, this chapter will cover bowel evacuation habits and laxative use.

Diet

A diet with adequate fiber is essential for decreasing constipation for most people. Fiber has other benefits to the body.

Basic Management of Constipation

Diet	25 to 35 grams of fiber per day 6 to 8 glasses of fluid per day
Exercise	15 to 30 minutes per day
Toileting	regular time
Habits	privacy sufficient time squatting position

Water soluble fibers help slow the absorption of glucose, a type of sugar, helping to improve blood sugar control in diabetics. Some fibers help lower blood cholesterol. Fiber may also help with weight loss because it increases the sense of being full, but doesn't add calories. High fiber foods also require more chewing, which slows the pace of eating.

North Americans typically have a diet that is very low in fiber, averaging 11 grams per day. The recommended daily amount of fiber is 25 to 35 grams, though the amount needed to prevent constipation can vary from person to person.

Sources of Fiber

The sources of fiber can be divided into two groups: insoluble and soluble. Insoluble fiber is found in fruit, vegetable skins, and the bran layer of wheat. Soluble fiber forms a gel in water. It is found in citrus fruit, cereals (e.g., barley, oatmeal, oat bran), and dried peas and beans. Not all fruits and vegetables are high in fiber. Beans, canned peas, broccoli, and raspberries are higher than most. Prunes are relatively high in fiber. The chart on page 152 lists some foods and their fiber content.

Eating at least four servings per day of fresh or cooked vegetables and fruits is a good base for getting enough fiber in the diet, as well as other essential nutrients. Adding 1 to 2 ounces of bran per day can be a simple way to increase overall fiber content.

Changing the diet is not always easy. Old habits die hard. Also, bran is not the most palatable food. It can be helpful to disguise it by adding it to meatloaf, cereal, muffins,

Foods and Their Fiber Content

Vegetables	Fiber	Fruit	Fiber
Asparagus, cooked	3.5	Apple	2.0
Green beans, cooked	2.1	Banana	1.5
Beets, cooked	2.1	Cranberries, $^1/_2$ c, raw	4.0
Broccoli, cooked	3.5	Melon	1.5
Cabbage, cooked	2.1	Orange	1.6
Carrots, raw	1.8	Peach	2.3
Lettuce, 1 c, fresh	0.8	Prunes, dried	2.8
Spinach, 1 c, fresh	0.2	Raisins, dried	1.0
Summer squash	2.0	Raspberries	4.6
Tomato, cooked/raw	1.5	Strawberries	2.3
Starchy Vegetables	**Fiber**	**Bread Fiber**	**Fiber**
Corn on the cob	2.6	Whole wheat	1.3
Green peas	6.7	Wheat bran, $^1/_2$ c, raw	12.0
Potato, baked	1.9	Popcorn, popped	3.0
Sweet potato	2.1	Rye flour	2.5
Cereals	**Fiber**	**Dried Peas/ Beans**	**Fiber**
All Bran	8.4	Brown beans	8.4
Corn Flakes	2.6	Kidney beans	9.7
Oat Bran	5.3	Pinto beans	8.9
Cheerios	2.5	Navy beans	7.9
Oatmeal	2.9	Lentils	3.7
Wheaties	2.6		

Note: These are approximate values for one serving of the food item. Fiber is given in grams.

Managing Constipation

applesauce, juices, or other foods. Visiting with a dietician can be helpful in sorting out what parts of a diet need to be changed and what are realistic ways to change it. It will also be important to make sure that teeth are in good condition to better break down foods as they enter the digestive system.

Fiber can cause some disturbing problems such as bloating, increased gas formation, stomache aches, and diarrhea, so it is important to add fiber very gradually, increasing the amount over several weeks. Usually such problems resolve over a 2 to 3 week period, after the body has adjusted to the increased fiber load. Caution should be used in adding fiber to the diet of someone who is bed-bound or who has a history of narrowing (strictures) in the intestine.

It is also important to have adequate fluid intake when adding fiber to the diet. Without adequate fluid intake, a high fiber diet can be constipating. This is discussed further in the next section. A proper diet with sufficient fiber and adequate fluids will ensure appropriate consistency of stool, without the need to resort to laxatives in most cases.

Fiber Supplements

Fiber supplements are sometimes necessary when diet alone is not controlling constipation. These are also called the "bulk-forming laxatives" which work by retaining water in the stool, thus increasing its bulk and stimulating the intestine to move along the contents. Examples of fiber supplements are:

Generic Name	Trade Name
methylcelluse	Citrucel®
psyllium	Metamucil®, Serutan®, Reguloid®
polycarbophil	Fibercon®

They can be taken one to three times a day, with their effect on the bowel occurring within 12 to 24 hours, although sometimes the full effect takes 2 to 3 days.

Fiber supplements can have the same side effects as fiber in foods and must be begun slowly and gradually increased. Some contain dextrose, a type of sugar, and should be avoided by diabetics. Sugar-free products are usually available. Some also contain salt (sodium) and should not be used by persons with congestive heart failure or persistent problems with too much fluid build-up in the body.

Homemade fiber recipes are available that work very well for many people. One method is to combine applesauce, prune juice, and bran in varying consistencies. This has been called "power pudding." An example is:

2 ^{1}/$_2$ cups applesauce

1 ^{1}/$_2$ cups prune juice

^{2}/$_3$ cups Allbran-type cereal

You can substitute 2 cups of diced pitted prunes for the prune juice and then blend the mixture. One tablespoon of the recipe can be mixed with orange juice. You can gradually increase up to 4 tablespoons per day. If you halve the amount of applesauce and prune juice, the recipe will have more of a pasty consistency and can be added to cereals or just eaten as is.

Another recipe is for "power balls." Use a ½ pound each of figs, dates, raisins, and prunes. Add one ounce of senna leaves (preferably preground). Grind all together in a food processor or meat grinder. Roll into 1-inch balls and serve at breakfast.

As with any addition of fiber, it is important to drink enough fluid. A good habit is to drink an additional glass of fluid at the time you take the supplement.

Fluid Intake

Poor fluid intake contributes to the formation of hard, dry stools that are difficult to evacuate. Since older persons tend to have a decreased perception of thirst, they are more likely than younger persons to have inadequate fluid intake. It is recommended that six to eight glasses of fluid per day is generally necessary to promote normal bowel function. If you have questions about how much fluid is appropriate for you to drink, ask your health care provider.

Exercise

Regular exercise is important for people because it keeps abdominal muscles in shape and helps stimulate the movement of stool through the large intestine. It can be very difficult to develop the habit of regular exercise, but it cannot only improve bowel function, but has many positive effects on health in general and overall sense of well-being.

Regular walking, 15 to 30 minutes per day, is an excellent exercise and usually one that most people can tolerate. Exercise programs that are done in a pool often work better for people with joint problems or arthritis. More aerobic exercise programs will probably require a medical examination to ensure adequate heart function.

Many chronic diseases of older persons result in the inability to do regular exercise. However, even simple stretching and strenghtening exercises of the arms or legs while sitting in a chair are beneficial and should be tried.

Toileting Habits

For any type of bowel problem, it is important to establish healthy bowel habits. A goal is for regular evacuation of the bowel, with "normal" ranging from three times per day to once every 3 to 5 days. To help establish this pattern, it is important to learn to respond to the urge to defecate when it comes, instead of putting it off to a more convenient time.

Setting aside a regular, private time and enough time to allow for complete evacuation is also important. You should allow at least 10 to 15 minutes, but no longer than 30 minutes. Sufficient time will also help you avoid straining with evacuation. Probably the best time is right after breakfast, taking advantage of the body's normal reflex to empty the bowel. The important thing is to find the time that works for you and then try to be consistent with that time.

You can actually train the bowel to a specific time by sitting on the toilet at the designated time, even if there is no urge to have a bowel movement. If repeated for several days, bowel function should gradually improve.

Being upright and in a squatting position over the toilet provides the best alignment for evacuation of the bowel. Most toilet seats are at a height to promote a squatting position. People requiring a raised toilet seat, which makes it easier to get up and down, can use a footstool to raise the knees and approximate squatting. Toilet comfort and safety should also be considered: a padded backrest and seat and handrails are some options available. Toilet substitutes can be used, such as commodes and bedpans, but care should be used to maintain privacy and proper positioning as much as possible.

Laxative Use

Laxatives include a wide variety of methods that help to empty the bowel. Laxatives should be used only after more natural methods have failed. Routine, long-term use should be avoided. In addition to the bulk-forming laxatives, which have already been discussed, there are four classes of laxatives: stimulants, saline cathartics, lubricants, and hyperosmotic laxatives. Examples of these laxatives are listed in the chart on page 158.

Stimulant Laxatives

Stimulant laxatives work by decreasing the loss of water from the bowel. They also can stimulate the wave-like motion in the bowel to move the contents along. Castor oil

Classification of Common Laxatives

Type	Generic Name	Trade Name
Bulk-forming	Methylcellulose	Citrucel®, Unifiber®
	Psyllium	Metamucil®, Serutan Reguloid®
	Polycarbophil	Fibercon®, Mitrolan®
Stimulant	Castor oil	
	Anthraquinones	Cascara Segrada®, Senn®, Aloe® Danthron®
Saline	Magnesium hydroxide	Milk of Magnesia®
	Magnesium citrate	Citrate of Magnesia®
	Sodium phosphate	
Lubricants	Docusate sodium	Colace®, Regutrol®
	Docusate calcium	
	Docusate potassium	
	Mineral oil	
Hyperosmotics	Lactulose	
	Sorbitol	
Suppositories	Bisacodyl	Dulcolax®
	Glycerine	
Enemas	Sodium phosphate	Fleet®
	Bisacodyl	Fleet®
	Mineral oil	Fleet®
	Docusate sodium	Therevac®

is a stimulant laxative, but it can damage the wall of the intestine and should not be used by older individuals. The anthraquinones (Cascara Segrada®, Senna®, Aloe®, Danthron®) are another type of stimulant which usually work in 6 to 8 hours. They can become habit forming, and long-term use can result in permanent loss of normal bowel function as in "cathartic colon," which is a colon that is featureless, enlarged, and sometimes shortened. These changes may not reverse once the stimulant is stopped. At times surgery is necessary to remove the damaged portion of the bowel.

Saline Cathartics

Saline cathartics are thought to pull fluid into the intestine through osmosis. They also stimulate the muscle activity of the intestinal wall. Examples are magnesium hydroxide (Milk of Magnesia®) and magnesium citrate (Citrate of Magnesia®). Results occur in 3 to 6 hours. They may cause imbalances in potassium, magnesium, or sodium (salt) levels and should not be used by persons with high magnesium or poor kidney function. Again, they are not indicated for long-term use.

Lubricants

Lubricants contain two classes. Stool softeners, such as docusate sodium (Colace®), make passage of stool easier by decreasing the surface tension of the fecal material so it can pick up more fluid. As with other laxatives, its use on a long-term basis should be avoided unless safer methods have failed, because there is some evidence that liver toxicity can occur with long-term use.

Mineral oil lubricates fecal matter and eases evacuation. Its use is generally avoided for elderly individuals, because of the risk of getting some into the lung when swallowing. Routine, regular use of mineral oil should also be avoided, because it can cause poor absorption of some vitamins.

Hyperosmotic Laxatives

Hyperosmotic laxatives stimulate the accumulation of fluid in the colon. They also increase acidity in the bowel, which improves motility. One type of hyperosmotic laxative is lactulose, which is a type of sugar. It passes unchanged into the colon, so it does not affect people with diabetes, and it is excellent to use for older individuals. It is safe to use with bed-bound persons or those with intestinal strictures. Another hyperosmotic laxative is sorbitol, which is a natural substance found in fruit and molasses. Effects on the bowel are seen 1 to 2 days after beginning the laxative.

Enemas

Enemas refer to a method of putting fluid into the rectum. The bulk of fluid stimulates evacuation by distending the rectal vault. Enemas are sometimes used to retrain the bowel to empty at regular intervals. They are available with solutions of all the different laxative types. Not more than 1 pint of fluid should be infused into the rectum. Care must be taken when inserting the

enema into the anus to avoid injury. Overuse should
be avoided.

Suppositories

Suppositories can also be placed into the rectum to stimulate evacuation. Bisacodyl (Dulocolax®) is a stimulant
laxative in tablet or suppository form. Glycerine suppositories work by drying the tissue in the rectum, producing
a reflex contraction to empty the bowel. Evacuation usually occurs in 15 to 30 minutes, though it can take up to 2
hours. Glycerine suppositories may cause rectal discomfort, irritation, and cramping.

Correct placement of a suppository is important. The
suppository should be placed in the anus and pushed
along the wall of the colon, beyond the internal and
external anal sphincters.

Summary

Many treatments for constipation can be used without
consulting a health care provider. Simple measures of
adequate fiber and fluid intake and exercise, as well as
good toileting habits, can often eliminate the problem.
Chronic constipation, however, should be evaluated by a
professional. If laxatives are needed on a frequent basis,
it will be important to seek help in finding ways to
restore more normal bowel function.

Chapter 12

Managing Fecal Incontinence

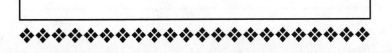

Fecal incontinence should never be considered normal aging. It can have many potential causes, as discussed in Chapter 9, and can respond to a variety of treatments. The treatment of fecal incontinence must fit the underlying factor(s) that are contributing to the problem. As mentioned earlier, gastrointestinal disorders may require specific treatment for infection, inflammatory disease, or cancer. Diarrhea can respond to antidiarrheal medication when appropriate, which works by increasing the resting pressure of the internal anal sphincter. Treatments and medications should be prescribed by your health care provider.

Fecal Impaction

As was mentioned in Chapter 9, severe constipation and partial blockage of the bowel is the most common cause of incontinence, because only soft or liquid stool gets around the blockage and can't be controlled as well.

Clearing the Bowel

The initial treatment for fecal impaction is to clear the bowel. This can be done with daily small bulk enemas until there is no return (usually 7 to 10 days). Sometimes it is necessary to manually remove the stool. With any possible impaction, a health care provider should be consulted for advice on causes and treatment.

Bowel Program

Once the bowel is clear, it is important to begin a bowel program in order to reestablish regularity. Adequate fiber and fluids in the diet, physical exercise as tolerated, and time to respond to the natural urge to defecate are important to diminish further constipation. You may also need a stool softener or osmotic laxative, as well as an enema or other bowel stimulant two to three times a week. These measures are discussed at length in the previous chapter. Your health care provider can help you decide which program might be best for you.

Habit Training

A related treatment for fecal impaction is a habit training program. This involves scheduling a specific time for toileting, generally right after breakfast when the normal urge to defecate tends to be the strongest. Measures to help habit training include providing adequate time and privacy to allow for evacuation. If no movement has occurred for 2 days, a small enema can be given. Gradually the bowel is retrained to the established pattern for defecation.

Structural Incontinence

Fecal incontinence that is due to a weakening of the pelvic floor muscles can sometimes respond to perineal exercises. Since the muscles involved extend from the anal area up past the bladder outlet, the same exercises for urinary incontinence are helpful. Perineal exercises can be augmented with the use of biofeedback. Both of these methods are described in Chapter 4.

Measures to avoid straining with defecation will also be important to prevent further structural changes that decrease bowel control. Maintaining normal consistency of stool is crucial. Refer to the previous section on constipation management for further explanation of these measures.

Neurogenic Incontinence

A bowel program can also be helpful for fecal incontinence resulting from problems with the nervous system. Ensuring normal stool consistency through regular exercise, adequate fluids, and fiber again is an essential first step. Persons with mental impairment often pass a formed stool once or twice a day. They still may sense the urge to evacuate, but are unable to stop it. It may be possible to note the typical times for defecation, and then help the person to the bathroom according to his or her pattern. The goal in toileting is to gradually increase the person's awareness of the urge to defecate.

Scheduled Toileting

Another method is to schedule toileting to occur 30 minutes after each meal. A stimulant suppository can be used initially to increase the person's awareness of the urge to defecate and to establish some consistency in evacuation. The use of a suppository can gradually be withdrawn as a regular pattern develops. A stimulant suppository works best with soft or already formed stool. For persons with severe mental impairment, it may be necessary to induce constipation for part of the day with an antidiarrheal agent and then stimulate evacuation with either a suppository or an enema. These programs should be discussed further with your health care provider.

Electrical Stimulation

In addition to basic bowel programs, there are other treatments that are available with some specialists in incontinence management. Electrical stimulation is being tried in attempts to increase perineal muscle tone and improve anal sphincter function. It is showing some success for fecal incontinence. There are different types of devices. One type has a probe that inserts into the rectum and gives a small electrical current. Another type has electrodes on small patches that stick to the skin around the anus. The electrical current stimulates the perineal muscles to contract. It works to strengthen the perineal muscle, thus improving bowel control. Results seem to be more successful when the person also does perineal muscle exercises along with the electrical stimulation. More information about electrical stimulation and perineal muscle exercises can be found in Chapter 4. However, further research is needed to better understand the benefits of using electrical stimulation for fecal incontinence.

Biofeedback

Biofeedback, discussed in Chapter 4, is another method that has shown up to a 63% success rate for fecal incontinence. Its use is beneficial with persons without mental impairment who are able to contract the external anal sphincter and who have some degree of rectal sensation. A probe is inserted into the rectum or electrodes are attached to the skin around the anus. The electrical current provided with contraction of the sphincters results in a visual and/or sound display. This gives the person information on the strength of the perineal muscle contraction. The person gradually increases the pressures exerted with sphincter contraction through subsequent sessions.

Anorectal manometry balloons can also be used for biofeedback. The balloon that is inserted into the rectum is filled with water to simulate increasing volume of stool. The individual is taught to tighten the external sphincter whenever filling is perceived in the rectum. Gradually the volume used to fill up the balloon is decreased so that the individual learns to respond to smaller and smaller volumes. The goal is to increase the person's ability to perceive rectal filling and to retain a certain volume.

Surgery

Several surgical procedures have been developed for treating fecal incontinence, especially when there is pelvic muscle relaxation and descent of the rectum. No single operation has proven to be the best. One surgical procedure tightens the anal canal with wires or elastic slings, but it is generally unsuccessful. Another surgery suspends the rectum back in its proper position and can increase bowel control in about two-thirds of persons. Sometimes removal of the rectum and sigmoid colon can be helpful, though often descent will reoccur. For a damaged anal sphincter, external sphincter repair is done. None of these procedures is free of complications, and sometimes the surgeons must construct a diverting colostomy before the actual repair work is done. A colostomy is when the bowel is brought out to the abdominal wall where a temporary opening is made for the evacuation of the bowel contents. Once the surgical area is repaired and healed, the bowel can be reattached in its proper position, and normal evacuation can resume.

There are many other surgical procedures available for specific problems of the bowel. It will be important for you to discuss these methods thoroughly with your health care provider or specialist, knowing the benefits and potential problems, before you proceed with this type of treatment.

Summary

Fecal incontinence is a common problem in older adults. It can have a variety of causes as well as treatments. A thorough evaluation by a health care provider will be helpful in finding the most appropriate management for the problem.

Chapter 13

Maintaining Dignity

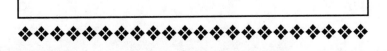

As mentioned in Chapter 2, not all incontinence can be cured. There are a group of individuals who for either physical and or medical reasons will always experience wetness. The goal for this group will then be to conceal and manage the incontinence. Developing a program which will enable the incontinent person to feel confident and secure with the containment of urine or stool will foster independence and socialization.

Therefore, this chapter will present information on the types of absorbant products available, controlling odor, skin care needs, suppliers, and suppport groups.

Selecting an Absorbant Product

In the past, incontinent products were poorly designed and seen merely as a larger version of a baby diaper or modification of a sanitary pad. Only recently have manufacturers placed a substantial investment into developing adult incontinent products that meet the needs of the users. The major function of absorbant products are to "soak up urine" for two reasons: (1) for the dignity of the user and (2) to protect clothing, furniture, bedding, and flooring (Brink, 1990).

Currently, there are at least 40 brand names of reusable and disposable products for adults on the market. These products include:

• Adult briefs (full garment with sticky tapes on either side to ensure a secure fit)

- Adult undergarments (full-length pad held in place by waist straps)

- Combination pad/pant systems

- Shields or pant liners

No one product will suit everyone. Many factors should be taken into consideration when choosing an absorbent pad or garment. For instance, the sex of the user, the type of incontinence (urine, stool, or both), mobility of the user, affordability of the product, disposability, and proximity of a retail outlet are all factors. In addition, the ideal product should meet the following criteria.

The product should:

- contain urine and/or stool completely without leakage onto clothing, furniture, or bedding,

- be comfortable to wear;

- prevent weakening and chaffing of the skin;

- easily concealed under clothing;

- be easy for the incontinent person and/or caregiver to get on and off; and

- contain odor.

Some brands of disposable absorbent pads and garments may be purchased at local shops, such as grocery, discount, pharmacies, and medical or home health stores. However, many products can be ordered directly from the manufacturer in bulk and delivered to the home. For more information on suppliers, refer to the section in this chapter on Service and Suppliers.

Adult Disposable Briefs

Because adults perceive wearing a "diaper" as degrading and embarrasing, you may find this product listed as an adult brief or underpant (see the illustration below). Most disposable briefs are made out of an absorbant polymer which, when it becomes wet, forms a gel and locks wetness in. Adult briefs come in several varieties. Most have elastic leg gathers to provide a snug fit. Others will also have elastic gathers at the waist. Some briefs have a wetness indicator. A wetness indicator is a colored

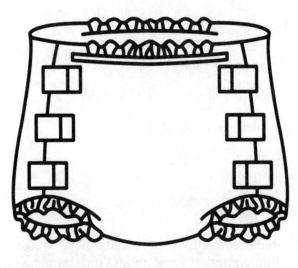

DEPEND® Fitted Briefs

Full adult brief.

strip that is on the outside of the garment. As leakage occurs, the colored strip becomes brighter or may change to a different color.

In general, characteristics of the disposable adult brief are:

• full brief that is secured by refastenable sticky tabs;

• intended for heavy leakage, can contain a full void;

• will contain both urine and stool;

• designed for men and women;

• will contain leakage when user is lying down;

• have a plastic backing; and

• are sized according to hip/waist measurement.

Cost of disposable briefs vary, and they are rarely reimbursed by insurance carriers.

Adult briefs are also available as reusables (see the illustration on page 176). Reusable briefs may be hourglass or retangular shape. Some brands have a built-in waterproof panel, whereas others must be used with a separate plastic pant. Reusable briefs require laundering on the hot water setting for two cycles to ensure proper disinfection. If laundering facilities are not available, or if the task of laundering is too difficult, other options exist. Some diaper services for infants also provide adult service. For a set monthly fee, the diaper service will provide the adult pad, the laundering, and the delivery of the product to the home.

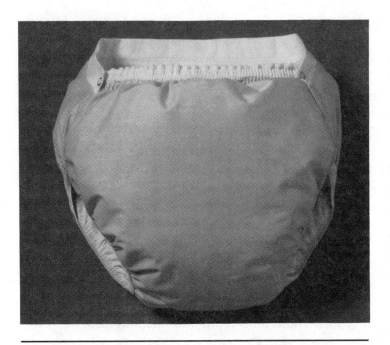

Reusable adult brief. (Courtesy of Dundee Mills Inc.)

When contacting a diaper service be specific about your needs. Questions to ask are:

- Does the service provide adult-size pads?

- Does the service provide a waterproof pant or do you have to purchase this item?

- What is their delivery schedule?

- What is the cost, and how does this compare to disposables?

Adult Undergarments

Adult undergarments are loincloth shaped pads that are
held in place by reusable elastic straps which button at
the waist (see the illustration below). Some undergarments are available with adjustable velcro straps which
may ease application for the person with limited hand
strength and mobility. Like adult briefs, the undergarments are made of a polymer for maximal absorption
without adding excessive bulk. Undergarments also are
available with and without elastic leg gathers.

Characteristics of the adult undergarment are:

• one-piece form-fitted pad with reusable straps to secure fit;

• intended for moderate to heavy urinary leakage;

• may be used with fecal incontinence, however, watery
  stools may not be contained;

• designed for users who are active and mobile;

• designed for men and women;

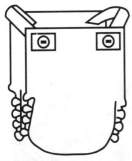
DEPEND® Undergarments
Elastic Leg

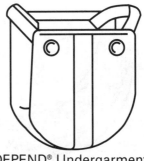
DEPEND® Undergarments
Non-Elastic Leg

Adult undergarments.

- sized according to hip/waist measurement; and

- not designed to contain wetness when lying down.

Cost of disposable undergarments vary, and cost is not reimbursed by insurance carriers.

Pad/Pant Systems

Pad/pant systems are designed to look and feel like underwear. The pant fits snugly to the body holding the pad in place thereby, increasing comfort, and providing minimal bulk. The pant is washable and the pads are disposable. The pad can either be a liner which is shaped like a sanitary pad (see the illustration below) or a full pad which could contain both urine and formed stool (see the illustration on page 179). The pads used with the pant system are all made of superabsorbant materials and can hold anywhere from 4 to 10 ounces or 120–300 cubic centimeters of urine.

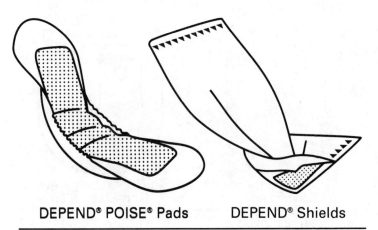

DEPEND® POISE® Pads   DEPEND® Shields

Liner.

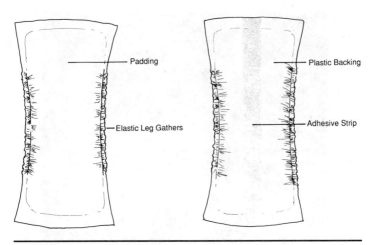

Large Liner.

There are many pad/pant systems available. Two of the more popular varieties are:

1. a full pad or small liner with a waterproof backing that is held in place with a cotton, jersey, or mesh pant (see the illustration on page 180),

2. a cotton or nylon pant that has plastic inner leg cuffs to protect for leakage (see the illustration on page 180). The pant is worn with a disposable liner.

For more information on product availability please refer to Appendix A.

Pant Liners

For many years men and women have used sanitary napkins to contain urine loss. Although somewhat absor-

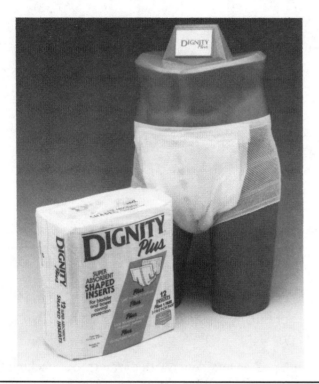

Mesh pad/pant system.

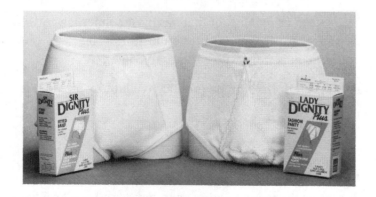

Nylon or cotton pad/pant system.

bant, sanitary pads do not offer odor control. There are many new pads available that have been specifically designed for urinary incontinence. Some of these liners are contoured to fit females (see the illustration on page 182), whereas others are shaped to cover the perineal area and buttocks offering increased protection and containment of formed stool (see the illustration on page 182).

General characteristics of the liners are:

• They are made of superabsorbants.

• They can be used for light to moderate leakage.

• They can be worn with regular underwear.

• They are secured to underpants by an adhesive strip.

• They have a waterproof backing.

• They are disposable.

Cost of the liners vary depending on the degree of protection: light, moderate, heavy.

There is also a specially designed liner for men. It is called a male drip collector (see the illustration on page 183). The drip collector is designed for men who have light urinary leakage or dribbling. The drip collector can hold up to 3 ounces or 90 cubic centimeters of urine. It is made of a superabsorbant material and has a waterproof backing. The drip collector must be worn with regular fitted underwear, athletic supporters, or a stretch mesh brief. The drip collector is held in place with an adhesive strip.

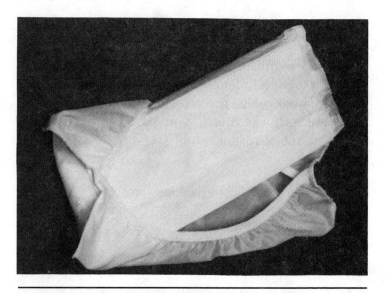

Small liner for pad/pant system.

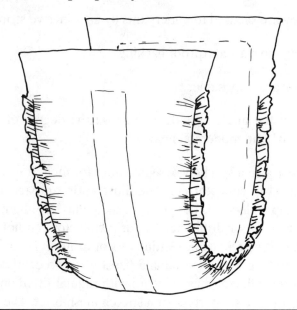

Large liner for pad/pant system.

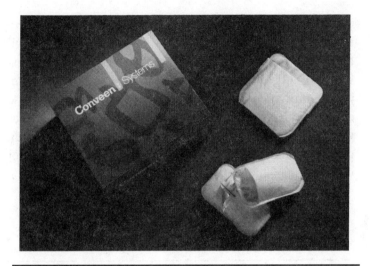

Male drip collector.

Controlling Odor

As mentioned earlier, using a pad designed for urinary incontinence will help control odor. In addition, room deodorizers or air fresheners are available to eliminate urine odor without leaving a lingering offensive scent rather than masking the smell.

An over-the-counter product can also be taken orally to help control odor. Chlorophyllin copper complex is a capsule which can be purchased without a prescription. Chlorophyll, when taken by capsule form, has been used as an internal deodorant for persons who have a colostomy (surgical opening made in the abdominal area to divert the emptying of bowel content into an external collecting bag).

The Federal Food and Drug Administration has recognized Chlorophyllin copper complex to be a safe and effective over-the-counter medication that can be used to reduce urine and stool odor. The dosage for Chlorophyllin complex is usually 100–200 milligrams per day. Excessive amounts of Chlorophyllin complex can cause abdominal cramps and diarrhea. Chlorophyllin complex will also change both urine and stool color to green. However, as with any medication, prescription or over the counter, please discuss this option with your health care provider before using Chlorophyllin complex.

Skin Care Needs

Urine and stool can be very damaging to skin. Both can produce redness and open sores which can be painful and increase the costs of incontinence management. Therefore, an important aspect of the incontinence management program needs to incorporate a skin care routine. Specially formulated skin care products are available to cleanse and protect skin exposed to urine and stool. A good skin care program should contain three steps: cleanse the skin, moisturize the skin, and protect the skin.

Cleansers

Incontinence cleansers allow for frequent washing of the skin without drying the skin out.

Characteristics of skin cleansers are:

- They dissolve urine and stool.

- They neutralize odor.

- They are nonirritating.

- They require no rinsing.

Cleansers are available in spray bottles, as foams, and in large pre-moistened towelettes which are disposable.

Moisturizers

Moisturizing creams for incontinence provide protection of the skin by hydrating it and by decreasing irritation and redness. Moisturizing creams should be rubbed in. If the cream is caked on, it can trap urine and stool and increase irritation to the skin. Moisturizing creams should be applied after each cleansing and especially when changing a soiled pad.

Barriers

Barrier creams or films act as a "second" skin and are used when damage has occured such as redness or open sores. Barrier creams are applied by gently rubbing the product on to the affected skin. Some creams need to be applied with each pad change. Barriers are also available as a spray or as a liquid which is "painted" onto the skin. In general, either product is applied only once a day and forms an invisible film over the skin. For most incontinent people, the cleansers and moisturizing creams will offer sufficient protection. For others, use of a barrier product may also be needed.

Discuss with your health care provider skin care product availability in your area. If your provider is not knowledgeable in product availability a medical supply or home health store should be able to provide you with the necessary information.

Service and Product Supply and Support Groups

As mentioned previously, many varieties of absorbant products are now available which are specially designed for the management of urine and stool loss. Although the assortment may be limited, some of these products can be purchased in local stores. Many major manufacturers, however, offer toll-free numbers, direct purchase, shipping, and someone to answer questions about the absorbant product you purchase. A list of manufacturers, addresses, and phone numbers can be found in Appendix A.

The American Association of Retired Persons publishes the AARP Pharmacy Services Catalog which offers a variety of incontinent products. Also incontinent supply companies have been formed solely to meet the needs of persons with incontinence. These companies offer a variety of products, a catalog which describes products available and cost, home delivery, and persons who can answer questions. Addresses and phone numbers of supply companies can be found in Appendix A.

National support groups have formed to meet the educational and emotional needs of persons with incontinence. Help For Incontinent People (HIP) is a nonprofit organization which provides information to the public and health care providers about the causes and treatment of incontinence. HIP publishes a quarterly newsletter which discusses treatment options, incontinent products, and an advisory column. HIP also publishes an incontinent resource guide which lists products and devices available for the management of incontinence and provides manufacturers addresses and phone numbers. In addition, HIP can help persons locate health care professionals in their areas who specialize in the assessment and management of incontinence.

The Simon Foundation and Continence Restored are similar organizations which offer printed information to the public and health professionals regarding the causes and treatment options available for incontinence. For addresses and phone numbers of support groups see Appendix B.

Summary

Incontinence is a problem that affects millions of Americans. For many, the leakage can be cured or substantially reduced. There are, however, persons who will always experience loss of urine or stool. For those individuals many new products have been developed to improve the containment of urine and stool. Support groups have also been formed to meet the educational and emotional needs of incontinent persons and their caregivers. As said many times throughout this book, the first step in treatment is a comprehensive evaluation to identify the cause of urine or stool loss. Reliance on an absorbant product for the management of incontinence should only occur after treatment options have been tried.

Appendix A

Products and Manufacturers

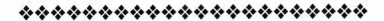

The listings in this appendix include both reusable and disposable absorbent products. The Manufacturers' Index includes address, phone numbers, and product name. Manufacturers are assigned a number. This number is listed next to the product in parentheses and can be used to find the manufacturers' information in the Manufacturers' Index. For example:

> 1.1 Absorbent Brief with Elastic Legs
>
> > Brand Name:
> > Attends (36)-manufacturer's number

Disposable Products

1.1 Absorbent Brief with Elastic Legs

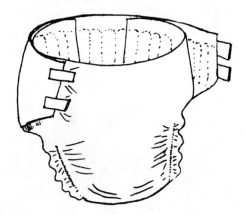

Brand Names:

At Ease (32)
Attends (55)
Assurance (13)
Bard (4)
Comfort Fit Plus (11)
Confidence (52)
Curity (37)
Depend (38)
Diaperbriefs (28)
Dignity Plus (33)
Dry Comfort (9)
First Quality (24)
Go Ahead (28)
Harmonie (9)
Kay Plus (16)
MaxiCare (47)
Natural (28)
Passport II (46)
Promise (58)
Protection Plus (48)
Prima Care II (57)
PrimeTime (47)
Provide (9)
PrimaCare II (57)
Reassure (30)
Secure (31)
Stanford (62)
SuretyS (15)
Skin-Caring (39)
Tranquility(53)
Ultigard (56)
UltraShield (65)
Wings(56)
Woodbury (66)
Woodbury Diaper
   Doubler (66)
Sears

1.2 Absorbent Brief Without Elastic Legs

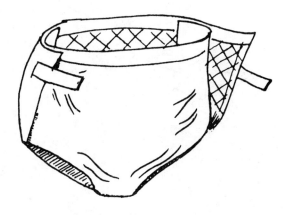

Brand Names:

Ables (27)
Ambeze (65)
Bard (4)
Bell-Horn (5)
Confidence
  Wingfold (52)
Curity (37)
Diaperbriefs (28)
Dignity Wingfold (33)
Duro-Med (19)
Go-Ahead (28)
Mark-Clark (23)

Medical Disposables (47)
Paper-Pak (30)
Passport (46)
PrimaCare I (57)
Protection Plus (48)
Stanford (62)
SureCare Wingfold (47)
Unigard II (56)
Val U Gard (56)
Woodbury (66)
Sears

1.3 Pad and Pant System

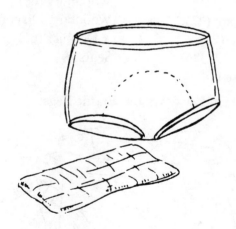

Brand Names:

At Ease (32)	Handicare (47)
Bell-Horn (5)	Hydas (35)
Confidence (52)	Lady Dignity Plus (33)
Curity (37)	Mark-Clark (23)
Dignity (17)	Nantucket (50)
Dignity Plus (33)	Safe and Dry (41)
DRIpride (9)	Salk-Knit (38)
Elderbrief (20)	Simplicity (47)
First Quality (24)	Sir Dignity Plus (33)
Free & Active (33)	Tranquility (53)
Geri-Care (15)	Revco

1.4 Absorbent Inserts—Flat

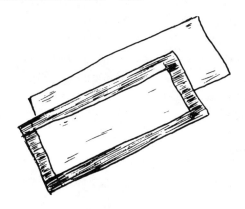

Brand Names:

ActivStyle (3)	Hospital Pack (14)
Aquagel (57)	Hydas (35)
Assurance (12)	Kay Plus (7)
At Ease (32)	Mark-Clark (23)
Attends (55)	Mark One (24)
Bell-Horn (5)	MaxiShield (65)
Breathe Easy (7)	MiniGard (65)
Buddies (46)	Perfer (57)
Confidence (52)	Promise (39)
Content I and II (9)	Protection Plus (48)
Curity (37)	Rejoice (7)
Curity (20)	Safe and Dry (41)
Dignity (33)	Secure (31)
DRIpride (9)	Securely Yours (30)
Dry Comfort (16)	Stanford (62)
Dura Tex (18)	Tape II (4)
Duro-Med (19)	Tranquility (34)
Elderbrief (20)	Tranquility (53)
Free and Active (33)	Unigard (56)
Freestyle (25)	Woodbury (66)
HandiCare (47)	Sears
Harmonie (9)	

1.5 Absorbent Inserts—Contoured

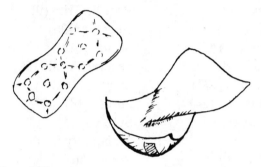

Brand Names:

Attends (55)	Poise Pads (38)
Confidence (52)	PrimaCare (57)
Curity (37)	Promise (58)
Depend (21)	Protection Plus (48)
Depend Shields (38)	Secure (31)
Dignity Plus Brief	Serenity (36)
Mates (33)	Simplicity (47)
Elderbrief (20)	Sure and Thin (47)
Full Life (60)	Surety (18)
Go-Ahead (14)	SuretyS (15)
Harmonie (9)	Woodbury (66)
Maxishield (65)	Sears

1.6 Undergarment

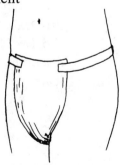

Brand Names:

At Ease (32)	Provide Trim (9)
Attends (55)	Reassure (30)
Carefor (57)	Secure (31)
Depend (38)	Securely Yours (52)
Dignity Plus (33)	Stanford (62)
First Quality (24)	Surety (18)
Full-Life (60)	SuretyS (15)
Hydas (35)	Tranquility (53)
MaxiCare (47)	Wings (56)
Protection Plus (48)	Woodbury (66)

1.7 Male Envelope-Style Drip Collector

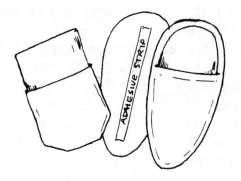

Brand Names:

Conveen (12)	Tranquility (34)
Go-Ahead (14)	Uri-Drain (40)
Harmonie (9)	Uro-Tex (41)
Manhood (59)	Woodbury (66)
Mentor (49)	Sears
Tenasorb (39)	

1.8 Male Gard

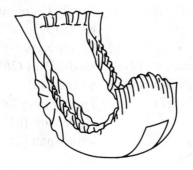

Brand Names:
Depend Guard (38)
Tranquility TrimShield (53)

Reusable Products

2.1 Diaper-Contoured

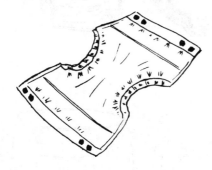

Brand Names:

Absorb-Plus (1)	Family Clubhouse (23)
Allstate (3)	KINS (39)
B-Dry (4)	Klassy Kare (40)
Comfort Concepts (14)	Med-I-Pant (26)
Confidentially Yours (11)	Softnit (48)
Dundee Mills (17)	The Wonder Diaper (64)
Edley (22)	Undercare (63)
Gabby's (26)	ValueSnap (2)
Geri-Care (29)	Sears

2.2 Reusable Brief

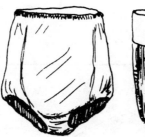
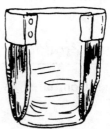

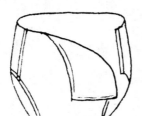
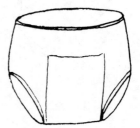

Brand Names:

ActivStyle (3)
Allstate (3)
Asorb-Plus (1)
A-T Surgical (1)
B-Dry (4)
Bell-Horn (5)
Biotechnics (6)
Camp Int'l. (6)
Carefor (57)
Comfort (13)
Comfort Concepts (14)
Confidentially Yours (11)
Curity (37)
Dignity (33)
DRIpride (9)
Dundee Mills (17)
DURA TEX (18)
Duro-Med (19)
Family Clubhouse (23)
Free & Active (33)
FreeStyle Maxi/Mini (25)
Geri-Care (29)
Handicare (47)
Hy-Tape (34)
Hydas (35)
KINS (39)
Klassy Kare (40)

Kloz-Ez (42)
Lady Dignity Plus (33)
Lifespan (2)
Mark-Clark (23)
MedI-Pant (26)
Maxishield (65)
Nantucket (50)
Nikky (29)
PCP Champion (51)
Pipeer (28)
Prefer (57)
Priva Acti-Fit (54)
Protection Plus (48)
Rejoice (7)
Rubber Duckies (37)
Safe and Dry (22)
Sani-Pant (57)
Sir Dignity Plus (33)
Soft & Silent (64)
Special Clothes
  Pull-On (61)
Tranquility (53)
Ultra Attends
  Pull-on (55)
Undercare (63)
ValueSnap (2)
Woodbury (66)
Sears

2.3 Mesh Stretch Brief

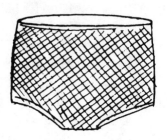

Brand Names:

Absorb-Plus (1)	Maintain (10)
Air-Flo (27)	Maintain Plus (10)
Assurance (12)	Maxishield (65)
Carefor (57)	Paper-Pak (30)
Cascade PSH (7)	Promise (58)
Conveen (12)	Protection Plus (48)
Curity (37)	Security (45)
Depend (21)	Woodbury (66)
DRIpride (9)	X-Span (2)
Easy-Brief (45)	K-Mart
Dispo-Brief (45)	Revco
Fancy-Free (45)	Sears
GEPCO (27)	

2.4 Contoured Liner

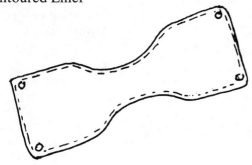

Brand Names:

Carefor (57)

Edley (22)

Freestyle (25)

Gabby's (26)

Geri-Care (29)

KINS (39)

Priva (54)

Sofnit (48)

2.5 Waterproof Pant

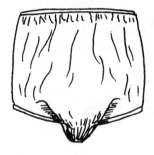 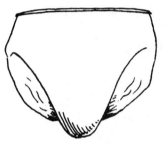

Brand Names:

ActivStyle (3)

Bell-Horn (5)

DURA TEX (18)

Edley (22)

Soft & Silent (64)

Special Clothes
Pull-On (61)

Undercare (63)

Woodbury (66)

2.6 Female Style Pant

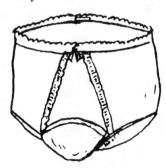

Brand Names:

ActivStyle (3)	Klassy Kare (40)
BreatheEasy (7)	Lady Dignity Plus (33)
Camp Int'l (8)	Nantucket (50)
Comfort (13)	Netti Flexi (43)
Danmar (16)	Premier (57)
E-Z Fit (21)	Safe and Dry (41)
Family Clubhouse (23)	Secure (31)
Free & Active (33)	SuretyS (15)
Geri-Care (29)	Undercare (63)
Hydas (35)	Woodbury (66)

2.7 Female Boxer-Style Pant

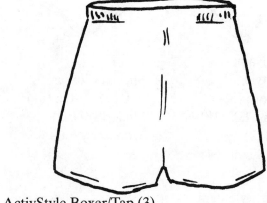

ActivStyle Boxer/Tap (3)

2.8 Men's Protective Support

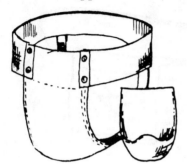

Klassy Kare (40)

2.9 Men's Fitted Brief

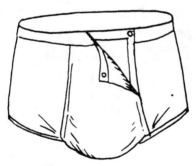

Brand Names:

ActivStyle (3)	Geri-Care (29)
BreatheEasy (7)	Nantucket (50)
Camp Int'l (8)	Netti Gentleman (43)
Comfort (13)	Prefer (57)
Danmar (16)	Premier (57)
Elderbrief (20)	Secure (31)
E-Z Fit (21)	Sir Dignity Plus (33)
Family Clubhouse (23)	Undercare (63)
Free & Active (33)	Woodbury (66)

2.10 Men's Drip Collector

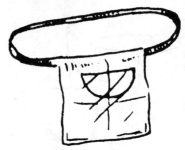

Brand Names:
Comfort (13)   Geri-Care (29)
Conveen (12)   Male Bag (44)

2.11 Men's Boxer Style Pant

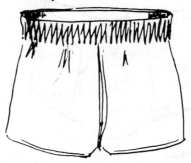

Brand Names:
ActivStyle (3)
Netti (43)
Security (45)

Adapted with permission from the *1994 HIP Resource Guide Products and Services For Incontinence.* The *HIP Resource Guide* is the most complete directory of products and services available. This directory of products and organizations assists people in finding the best management solutions.

Manufacturer's Index

1. A-T Surgical Mfg. C., Inc.
115 Clemente Street
Holyoke, MA 01040
413-532-4551
413-532-0826 (fax)
800-225-2023

2.2 Reusable Brief

2. Allstate Medical Products, Inc.
14001 Ridgedale Drive
Suite 330
Minnetonka, MN 55305-1783
612-541-0506
612-541-0558 (fax)
800-328-2915

2.1 ValueSnap reusable adult diaper
2.2 ValueSnap reusable adult brief

3. American Health Products
5353 Wayzata Blvd.
Suite 615
Minneapolis, MN 55305-1783

612-544-6223
612-544-0680 (fax)
800-651-6223

1.4 ActivStyle disposable flat insert
2.2 ActivStyle reusable brief
2.5 ActivStyle waterproof pant

2.6   ActivStyle female style pant
    2.7   ActivStyle female boxer style pant
    2.9   ActivStyle men's fitted brief
    2.11 ActivStyle men's boxer style pant

4. B-Dry
2307 Bellmore Avenue
Bellmore, NY 11710
516-826-3482 (fax)
800-826-BDRY (800-826-2379)

    2.1 Reusable diaper
    2.2 Reusable brief

5. Bell-Horn
(William H. Horn & Brothers, Inc.)
451 North Third Street
Philadelphia, PA 19123-4197
215-627-2773
800-366-4676

    1.2 Disposable brief
    1.3 Pad-and-pant starter kit
    1.4 Absorbent insert-flat
    2.5 Waterproof pant

6. Biotechnics Management Ltd.
2038 East 3110 South
P.O. Box 9407
Salt Lake City, UT 84109
801-484-6833
801-486-9903 (fax)

    2.2 Reusable brief

7. C.P. International, Inc.
250 Park Avenue, Suite 1930
New York, NY 10177
212-599-288
212-687-0248 (fax)

1.4 BreatheEasy absorbent inserts-flat
2.2 Rejoice reusable brief
2.6 BreatheEasy female style pant
2.9 BreatheEasy men's fitted brief

8. Camp International, Inc.
P.O. Box 89
Jackson, MI 49204
517-787-1600
517-789-3299 (fax)
800-492-1088

2.6 Female style pant
2.9 Men's fitted brief

9. Cascade H.B.A., Inc.
First Street
Palmer. MA 01069-0720
413-289-1221
413-289-1367 (fax)
800-666-1205

1.1 Dry Comfort absorbent brief
1.1 Harmonie adult brief
1.4 Harmonie absorbent insert-flat
1.5 Harmonie absorbent insert-contoured
1.7 Harmonie male envelope-style drip collector

10. Cascades P.S.H., Inc.
999 Farrel
Drummondville, Quebec
Canada J2C-5P6
819-477-5077
819-477-8779 (fax)
800-567-0692 (only in Canada)

2.3 Maintain mesh stretch brief
2.3 Maintain Plus mesh stretch brief

11. Clinitex Holdings, Inc.
9801 Kincey Avenue, Suite 190
Huntersville, NC 28078
704-875-0806
704-875-0810 (fax)

1.1 Comfort Fit-Plus adult brief

12. Coloplast, Inc.
5610 W. Sligh Avenue
Tampa, Fl 33634
813-885-4213 (fax)
800-237-4555

1.7   Conveen envelope-style drip collector
2.3   Conveen mesh brief
2.10 Conveen male drip collector

13. Comfort
377 Bering Avenue
Toronto, Ontario
Canada M8Z-3B1

416-763-6740
416-604-3722 (fax)
800-463-2217

1.2 Comfort absorbent brief
2.2 Comfort reusable brief
2.6 Comfort female style pant
2.9 Comfort men's fitted brief
2.10 Comfort men's drip collector

14. Comfort Concepts, Inc.

114 Essex Street
Rochelle Park, NJ 07662
201-368-2448
201-368-2457 (fax)
800-935-2241

2.1 Comfort Concepts reusable diaper
2.2 Comfort Concepts reusable brief

15. Confab (ICD Industries)

601 Allendale Road
King of Prussia, PA 19406
610-337-7200
610-337-3908 (fax)
800-262-0042

1.1 SuretyS adsorbent adult brief
1.5 SuretyS absorbent insert-contoured
1.6 SuretyS adult undergarment
2.6 SuretyS female style pant

16. Danmar Products, Inc.
221 Jackson Industrial Drive
Ann Arbor, MI 48103
313-761-1990
313-761-8977 (fax)
800-783-1998

2.6 Danmar female style pant
2.9 Danmar men's fitted brief

17. Dundee Mills, Inc.
111 West 40th Street
New York, NY 10018
212-840-7200
212-840-3980 (fax)

2.1 Reusable diaper
2.2 Reusable brief

18. DURA TEX
P.O. Box 67, Dept. 315
Leipsic, OH 45856
419-943-2315
800-628-4761

1.4 DURA TEX adsorbent inserts-flat
2.2 DURA TEX reusable brief
2.5 DURA TEX waterproof pant

19. Duro-Med Industries, Inc.
155 Polifly Road
Hackensack, NJ 07602

201-488-5055
201-488-6212 (fax)
800-526-4753

1.2 Duro-Med adsorbent adult brief
1.4 Duro-Med absorbent inserts-flat
2.2 Duro-Med reusable brief

20. Elderbrief

402 East Charles Street
P.O. Box 682
Bryan, OH 43506
419-636-7887
419-636-7893 (fax)
800-466-6646

1.3 Elderbrief pad/pant system
1.4 Elderbrief absorbent inserts-flat
1.5 Elderbrief absorbent inserts-contoured
2.9 Elderbrief men's fitted brief

21. E-Z- Fit Corporation

53-16 62nd Street
Maspeth, NY 11378
718-507-6664

2.6 Female style pant
2.9 Men's fitted brief

22. Edley Enterprises, Inc.

P.O. Box 429
Sanbornville, NH 03872-0429
603-473-2539

2.1 Reusable diaper
2.4 Contoured liner
2.5 Waterproof pant

23. Family Clubhouse, Inc.
6 Chiles Avenue
Asheville, NC 28803
704-254-9236
704-258-9052 (fax)
800-876-1574

2.1 Reusable diaper-countoured
2.2 Reusable brief
2.6 Female style pant
2.9 Men's fitted brief

24. First Quality Products, Inc.
80 Cutter Mill Road, Suite 409
Great Neck, NY 11021
516-829-3030
516-829-4949 (fax)
800-488-3130

1.1 First Quality absorbent brief
1.3 First Quality pad/pant system
1.6 First Quality undergarment

25. Freestyle Medical Supplies, Inc.
336 Green road
Stoney Creek, Ontario
Canada L8E-2B2

905-662-4281
905-662-8723 (fax)
800-841-5330

1.4 Freestyle absorbent inserts-flat
2.2 Freestyle reusable brief
2.4 Freestyle contoured liner

26. Gabby's
386 Hendoon Drive NW
Calgary, Alberta
Canada T2K-2Z7
403-282-8503
403-282-8503 (fax)

2.1 Contoured diaper
2.4 Contoured liner

27. General Econpak, Inc.
(GEPCO)
1725 North Sixth Street
Philadelphia, PA 19122
215 763-8200

2.3 GEPCO mesh brief

28. George Disposables
2221 Peachtree Road
Suite D
Atlanta, GA 30309
404-350-9410
404-350-9416 (fax)
800-950-3427

1.1 Diaperbriefs absorbent brief with elastic legs
1.1 Go-Aheads absorbent brief with elastic legs
1.1 Natural absorbent brief with elastic legs
1.2 Diaperbriefs absorbent brief without elastic legs
1.2 Go Aheads absorbent brief without elastic legs

29. Geri-Care Products
252 Wagner Street
Middlesex, NJ 08846
908-469-7722
908-469-9473(fax)

2.1   Contoured diaper
2.2   Reusable brief
2.4   Contoured liner
2.6   Female style pant
2.9   Men's fitted brief
2.10 Men's drip collector

30. Home Delivery Incontinent Supplies Co., Inc. (HDIS)
1215 Dielman Industrial Court
Olivette, MO 63132
314-997-8771
314-997-0047 (fax)
800-538-1036

1.1 Reassure absorbent brief
1.6 Reassure undergarment

31. G. Hirsch & Company, Inc.
1525 Adrian Road
Burlingame, CA 94010

415-692-8770
415-692-1874 (fax)
800-632-7960

1.1 Secure absorbent brief
1.4 Secure absorbent inserts-flat
1.5 Secure absorbent inserts-contoured
1.6 Secure undergarment
2.6 Secure female style pant
2.9 Secure men's fitted brief

32. Hospital Specialty Company

7501 Carnegie Avenue
Cleveland, OH 44103
216-361-1230
216-361-0829 (fax)
800-B-AT-EASE (800-228-3273)

1.1 At Ease Absorbent brief
1.3 At Ease pad/pant system
1.4 At Ease absorbent inserts-flat
1.6 At Ease undergarment

33. Humanicare International, Inc.

1200 Airport Road
P.O. Box 1939
North Brunswick, NJ 08902
201-214-0660
800-631-5270

1.1 Dignity Plus absorbent brief
1.2 Dignity Wingfold absorbent brief
1.3 Dignity pad and pant
1.3 Free & Active pad and pant system

1.3 Sir Dignity Plus pad and pant system
1.3 Lady Dignity Plus pad and pant system
1.4 Dignity absorbent insert-flat
1.4 Free & Active absorbent insert-flat
1.5 Dignity Plus Brief Mates absorbent inserts-
       contoured
1.6 Dignity Plus undergarment
2.2 Dignity reusable brief
2.2 Free & Active reusable brief
2.2 Lady dignity Plus reusable brief
2.2 Sir Dignity Plus reusable brief
2.6 Free & Active female style pant
2.6 Lady dignity Plus female style pant
2.9 Free & Active men's fitted brief
2.9 Sir Dignity Plus men's fitted brief

34. Hy-Tape Surgical Products Corp.
772 McLean Avenue
Yonkers, NY 10704
914-237-1234
914-237-7267 (fax)
800-248-0101

2.2 Reusable brief

35. Hydas, Inc.
P.O. Box 420
Hershey, PA 17933
717-533-5583
717-533-5548 (fax)
800-358-5583

1.3 Hydas pad/pant system
1.4 Hydas absorbent insets-flat

1.6 Hydas undergarment
2.2 Hydas reusable brief
2.6 Hydas female style pant

36. Personal Products Company

Johnson & Johnson
Van Liew Avenue
P.O. Box 900
Milltown, NJ 08850
908-524-0500
908-524-0045 (fax)
800-526-3967

1.5 Serenity guards

37. Kendall-Futuro Company

Suite A, 5405 Dupont circle
Cincinnati, OH 45150
513-576-8000
513-576-8273 (fax)
800-543-4452

1.1 Curity contoured brief
1.2 Curity adult brief
1.3 Curity pad and pant system
1.4 Curity liner
1.5 Curity shield
2.2 Curity reusable brief
2.3 Curity mesh brief

38. Kimberly-Clark, Corp.
2001 Marathon Avenue
Neenah, WI 54956
800-558-6423

1.1 Depend fitted brief
1.5 Depend shields
1.5 Proise Pads
1.6 Depend undergarment
1.8 Depend Guard

39. Kinder Incontinent Supplies (KINS)
#4-3531 Jacombs Road
Richmond, B.C.
Canada, V6V-1Z8
604-270-6116
604-270-2124 (fax)
800-665-2229

2.1 KINS reusable diaper
2.2 KINS reusable brief
2.4 KINS contoured liner

40. Klassy Kare
P.O. Box 229
Glyndon. MN 56547
218-498-2544

2.1 Klassy Kare reusable diaper
2.2 Klassy Kare reusable brief
2.6 Klassy Kare female style pant
2.8 Klassy Kare men's protective support

41. Kleinert's Inc.

120 W. Germantown Avenue
Suite 100
Plymouth Meeting, PA 19462
215-828-7261
215-828-4589 (fax)

1.3 Safe and Dry pad and pant system
1.4 Safe and Dry absorbent insert-flat
2.6 Safe and Dry female style pant

42. Kloz-Ez

1065-D Shary Circle
Concord, CA 94518
510-689-1316
510-689-0705 (fax)
800-848-5540

2.2 Kloz-Ez reusable brief

43. LL Medico U.S.A., Inc.

1512 West Chester Pike #255
West Chester, PA 19382
610-436-8831
610-436-4537 (fax)

2.6   Netti Flexi female style pant
2.9   Netti Gentleman men's fitted brief
2.11 Netti men's boxer style pant

44. Longstreet Pharmacal Corporation

1218 50th Street
Brooklyn, NY 11219

718-436-9200
718-854-2431 (fax)
800-633-7878

2.10 Male Bag men's drip collector

45. MB Products, Ltd.
120 Swannanoa River Road
Asheville, NC 28805
704-253-8874
704-254-4269 (fax)

2.3   Easy-Brief mesh stretch brief
2.3   Dispo-Brief mesh stretch brief
2.3   Fancy free mesh stretch brief
2.3   Security mesh stretch brief
2.11 Security men's boxer style pant

46. Mark One Healthcare Products
Div. of Struble and Moffitt Company
P.O. Box 263
100 East Ninth Avenue
Runnemede, MJ 08078
609-939-5400
609-939-4187 (fax)
800-631-3549

1.1 Passport II absorbent brief
1.2 Passport adult brief
1.4 Buddies absorbent insert-flat

47. Company
1165 Hayes Industrial Drive
Marietta, GA 30062
404-422-3036
404-427-6632 (fax)
800-241-8205

1.1 MaxiCare fitted brief
1.1 PrimeTime contoured brief
1.2 Medical Disposables absorbent brief
1.2 SureCare Wingfold absorbent brief
1.3 HandiCare pad and pant system
1.3 Simplicity pad and pant system
1.4 HandiCare absorbent insert-flat
1.5 Sure and Thin absorbent insert-contoured
1.5 Simplicity absorbent insert-contoured
1.6 MaxiCare undergarment
2.2 HandiCare reusable brief

48. Medline Industries, Inc.
One Medline Place
Mundelein, IL 60060
708-949-5500
708-949-3189 (fax)
800-289-9793

1.1 Protection Plus absorbent brief
1.2 Protection Plus absorbent brief
1.4 Protection Plus absorbent insert-flat
1.5 Protection Plus absorbent insert-contoured
1.6 Protection Plus undergarment
2.1 Sofnit reusable diaper
2.2 Protection Plus reusable brief

2.3 Protection Plus mesh stretch brief
2.4 Sofnit contoured liner

49. Mentor

5425 Hollister Avenue
Santa Barbara, CA 93111
805-681-6000
805-681-6166 (fax)
800-328-3863

1.7 Mentor male envelope-style drip collector

50. Nantucket Industries, Inc.

195 Madison Avenue
New York, NY 10016
212-889-5656
212-532-3217 (fax)
800-562-3774

1.3 Nantucket pad and pant system
2.2 Nantucket reusable brief
2.6 Nantucket female style pant
2.9 Nantucket men's fitted brief

51. PCP-Champion

300 Congress Street
Ripley, OH 45167
513-392-4301
800-888-0867 (fax)
800-888-0458

2.2 Reusable brief

52. Paper-Pak Products, Inc.
1941 White Avenue
LaVerne, CA 91750
909-392-1200
909-392-1204 (fax)
800-635-4560

1.1 Confidence absorbent brief
1.2 Confidence Wingfold absorbent brief
1.5 Confidence absorbent insert-contoured
1.6 Securely Yours undergarment

53. Principle Business Enterprises, Inc.
Pine Lake Industrial Park
Dunbridge, OH 43414
419-352-1551
419-352-8340 (fax)
800-467-3224

1.1 Tranquility SlimLine underpant
1.3 Tranquility pad and reusable brief
1.4 Tranquility flat shield
1.6 Tranquility undergarment
1.8 Tranquility TrimShield male gard
2.2 Tranquility reusable brief

54. Priva, Inc.
P.O. Box 448
Champlain, NY 12919-0048
514-356-0055 (fax)
800-361-4964

2.2 Priva reusable brief
2.4 Priva contoured liner

55. Proctor & Gamble Company
P.O. Box 599
Cincinnati, OH 45201
800-543-0480

1.1 Attends absorbent brief
1.3 Ultra Attends pad and pant system
1.4 Attends absorbent insert-flat
1.5 Attends absorbent insert-contoured
1.6 Attends undergarment
2.2 Ultra Attends Pull-on reusable brief

56. Professional Medical Products
P.O. Box 3288
Greenwood, SC 29648
803-223-4281
803-229-9129 (fax)
800-845-4571

1.1 Wings fitted brief
1.1 Ultigard fitted brief
1.2 Unigard II disposable brief
1.2 Val U Gard absorbent brief
1.4 Unigard flat insert
1.6 Wings undergarment

57. Salk Company, Inc.
P.O. Box 452
119 Braintree Street
Boston, MA 02134
617-782-4030
617-782-9402 (fax)
800-343-4497

1.1 PrimaCare II fitted brief
1.2 PrimaCare I brief
1.4 Aquagel flat insert
1.4 Prefer flat insert
1.5 PrimaCare absorbent insert-contoured
1.6 Carefor undergarment
2.2 Carefor reusable brief
2.2 Prefer reusable brief
2.2 Sani-Pant reusable brief
2.3 Carefor mesh stretch brief
2.4 Carefor contoured liner
2.6 Premier female style pant
2.9 Prefer men's fitted brief
2.9 Premier men's fitted brief

58. Scott Health Care Products
Scott Plaza
Philadelphia, PA 19113
800-992-9939

1.1 Promise absorbent brief
1.5 Promise contoured insert
2.3 Promise mesh brief

59. Sierra Laboratories, Inc.
3520 South Campbell
Tuscon, AZ 85713
602-624-0580
602-624-0598 (fax)
800-726-2904

1.7 ManHood male envelope-style drip collector

60. Simera Corporation
1525 Adrian Roan
Bulingame, CA 94010
415-692-6980

1.5 Full Life absorbent inserts-contoured
1.6 Full Life undergarments

61. Special Clothes
P.O. Box 4220
Alexandria, VA 22303
703-683-7343
703-549-2640 (fax)

2.2 Special Clothes Pull-On Reusable brief
2.5 Special Clothes Pull-On waterproof pant

62. Stanford Professional Products Corp.
1416 Union Avenue
Pennsauken, NJ 08110
609-665-4054
609-665-3511 (fax)
800-345-3929

1.1 Stanford absorbent brief
1.2 Stanford absorbent brief
1.4 Stanford absorbent insert-flat
1.6 Stanford undergarment

63. Undercare
Div. of Visa Therm Products, Inc.
P.O. Box 486
Bridgeport, CT 06604

203-334-4560
203-334-5012 (fax)

2.1 Undercare reusable diaper
2.2 Undercare reusable brief
2.5 Undercare waterproof pant
2.6 Undercare female style pant
2.9 Undercare men's fitted pant

64. Vinyl Incontinent Products, Inc.
P.O. Box 63
Three Oaks, MI 49128
616-756-7382

2.1 The Wonder Diaper reusable diaper
2.2 Soft & Silent reusable brief
2.5 Soft & Silent waterproof pant

65. Whitestone Products
40 Turner Place
Piscataway, NJ 08854
908-752-2700
908-752-3984 (fax)
800-526-3567

1.1 UltraShield fitted brief
1.2 Ambeze incontinent pant
1.4 MaxShield flat insert
1.4 MiniGard flat insert
1.5 MaxiShield absorbent insert-contoured
2.2 Maxishield reusable brief
2.3 Maxishield mesh brief

66. Woodbury Products, Inc.
4410 Austin Blvd.
Island Park, NY 11558
516-431-6793 (fax)
800-879-3427
800-777-1111

1.1 Woodbury absorbent brief
1.1 Woodbury Diaper Doubler absorbent brief
1.2 Woodbury absorbent brief
1.3 Woodbury pad and pant system
1.4 Woodbury absorbent insert-flat
1.5 Woodbury absorbent inset-contoured
1.6 Woodbury undergarment
1.7 Woodbury male envelope-style drip collector
2.2 Woodbury reusable brief
2.3 Woodbury mesh stretch brief
2.5 Woodbury waterproof pant
2.6 Woodbury female style pant
2.9 Woodbury men's fitted brief

Adapted with permission from the HIP foundation, 1994 Resource Guide.

Appendix B

Self-Help Groups
and Agencies

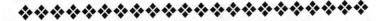

Agency for Health Care Policy and Research
P.O. Box 8547
Silver Spring, Maryland 20907
800-358-9295

Alliance for Aging Research
2021 K Street NW
Suite 305
Washington, DC 20006
202-293-2856

American Foundation for Urologic Disease
300 West Pratt Street, Suite 401
Baltimore, Maryland 21201
401-727-2908
800-242-2383

American Society on Aging
833 Market Street, Suite 512
San Francisco, CA 94103
415-543-2617

Association of Rehabilitation Nurses
2506 Gross Point Road
Evanston, IL 60201
312-475-7300

Continence Restored, Inc.
407 Strawberry Hill
Stanford, CT 06905
212-879-3131 (Daytime)
203-348-0601 (Evening)

HIP (Help for Incontinent People)
P.O. Box 544
Union, SC 29379
803-579-7900

National Institue On Aging
National Institutes of Health
Federal Building, Room 6C12
Bethesda, MD 20892
301-496-1752

National Kidney Foundation
30 E. 33rd Street
New York, NY 10016
800-622-9010

National Kidney and Urologic Diseases
Information Clearinghouse
P.O. Box NKUDIC
Bethesda, MD 20892
301-468-6345

National Spinal Cord Injury Association
369 Elliot Street
Newton Upper Falls, MA 02164
617-964-0521

Simon Foundation
P.O. Box 815
Wilmette, IL 60091
800-23SIMON

Simon Foundation Canada
P.O. Box 3221
Tecumseh, Ontario N8N 2M4
Canada
800-265-9575

Adapted with permission from the 1994 HIP Resource Guide Products and Services For Incontinence

The HIP Resource Guide is the most complete directory of products and services available. This directory of products and organizations assists people in finding the best management solutions.

References

Barrett, J. (1990). Treating fecal incontinence. *Nursing Times, 86*(30), 66–70.

Brink, C. A. (1990.) Absorbant pads, garments, and management strategies. *Journal of the American Geriatric Society, 38*(3), 368–373.

Burgio, K. L., & Engel, B. T. (1990). Biofeedback-assisted behavioral training for elderly men and women. *Journal of the American Geriatric Society, 38*(3), 338–340.

Burgio, K. L., Pearce, K. L., & Lucco, A. J. (1989). *Staying Dry*. Baltimore: The John Hopkins University Press.

Folstein, M. F., Folstein, S., & McHugh, P. R. (1975). Mini-mental state: A practical method for grading the cognitive state of patients for the clinician. *Journal of Psychiatric Research, 12,* 189–198.

Goldstein, M. K., Brown, E. M., Holt, P, Gallagher, D. & Winograd, C. H. (1989). Fecal incontinence in an elderly man. *Journal of the American Geriatric Society, 37*(10), 991–1002.

Gray, M. L. (1990). Assessment and investigation of urinary incontinence. In K. Jeter, N. Fuller, & C. Norton, (Eds), *Nursing for continence* (pp. 25–36). Philadelphia: W. B. Saunders.

Hammon, T. P. The development of continence and causes of incontinence. In K. Jeter, N. Fuller, & C. Norton, (Eds), *Nursing for continence* (pp. 9–13). Philadelphia: W. B. Saunders.

Herzog A. R., & Fultz, N. H. (1990). Prevalence and incidence of urinary incontinence in community-dwelling populations. *Journal of the American Geriatric Society, 38*(3), 273–281.

Jeter, K. (1990). The use of incontinence products. In K. Jeter, N. Fuller, & C. Norton, (Eds), *Nursing for continence* (pp. 209–220). Philadelphia: W. B. Saunders.

Kane, R. L., Ouslander, J. G., & Abrass, I. B. (1989). Essentials of clinical geriatrics. New York: McGraw-Hill.

Mahoney, F. I., & Barthel, D. W. (1965). Functional evaluation: the barthel index. *Maryland State Medical Journal, 14,* 61–65.

McDowell, B. J., Burgio, K. L., & Candib, D. (1990). Behavioral and pharmacological treatment of persistent urinary incontinence in the elderly. *Journal of the American Academy of Nurse Practitioners, 2*(1), 17–23.

Morishita, L. S. (1987). The management of urinary incontinence by community-living elderly. *The Gerontologist, 27*(2), 185–193.

National Institutes of Health Consensus Conference. (1989). Urinary incontinence in adults. *JAMA, 261*(18), 2685–2690.

Pires, M. (1990). Promoting continence for the physically impaired. In K. Jeter, N. Fuller, & C. Norton, (Eds), *Nursing for continence* (pp. 159–167). Philadelphia: W. B. Saunders.

Plamer, M. H. (1990). Incontinence in the elderly. In K. Jeter, N. Fuller, & C. Norton, (Eds), *Nursing for continence* (pp. 139–153). Philadelphia: W. B. Saunders.

Read, N. W., & Timms, J. M. (1986). Defecation and the pathophysiology of constipation. *Clinics in Gastroenterology, 15*(4), 937–965.

Rousseau, P. (1990). Managing constipation in the elderly patient. *Family Practice Recertification, 12*(5), 76–95.

Schiller, L. R. (1986). Feacal incontinence. *Clinics in Gastroenterology, 15*(3), 687–704.

Stone, J. T. (1991). Managing bowel function. In W. C. Chenitz, J. T. Stone, & S. A. Salisbury (Eds), *Clinical gerontological nursing* (pp. 217–232). Philadelphia: W. B. Saunders.

Tanagho, E. A. (1990). Electrical stimulation. *Journal of the American Geriatric Society, 38*(3), 352–355.

Wald, A. (1986). Fecal incontinence: Effective nonsurgical treatments. *Postgraduate Medicine, 80*(3), 123–130.

Wells, T. J. (1990). Pelvic (floor) muscle exercises, *Journal of the American Geriatric Society, 38*(3), 333–337.

Whitehead, W. E., Drinkwater, D, Cheskin, L. J., Heller, B. R., & Schuster, M. M. (1989). Constipation in the elderly living at home. *Journal of the American Geriatric Society, 37*(5), 423–429.

Wyman, J. (1988). Nursing assessment of the incontinent geriatric outpatient population. *Nursing Clinics of North America, 23*(1), 169–187.

Wyman, J. F. (1991). Incontinence and related problems. In W. C. Chenitz, J. T. Stone, & S. A. Salisbury (Eds), *Clinical gerontological nursing* (pp. 192–201). Philadelphia: W. B. Saunders.

Index